NEUROTRANSMITTER RECEPTOR BINDING

Neurotransmitter Receptor Binding

Editors:

Henry I. Yamamura, Ph.D.
Associate Professor
Department of Pharmacology
College of Medicine
The University of Arizona Health Sciences Center
Tucson, Arizona

S. J. Enna, Ph.D.
Associate Professor
Departments of Pharmacology and Neurobiology and Anatomy
The University of Texas Medical School at Houston
Houston, Texas

Michael J. Kuhar, Ph.D.
Associate Professor
Departments of Pharmacology and Psychiatry
The Johns Hopkins University School of Medicine
Baltimore, Maryland

Raven Press ▪ New York

Raven Press, 1140 Avenue of the Americas, New York, New York 10036

Made in the United States of America

Library of Congress Cataloging in Publication Data

Neurotransmitter receptor binding.

Includes bibliographical references and index.
1. Neurotransmitters–Analysis. 2. Neurotransmitter receptors. 3. Radioligand assay.
I. Yamamura, Henry I. II. Enna, S. J.
III. Kuhar, Michael J. [DNLM: 1. Neurohumors.
2. Synaptic receptors. 3. Binding sites.
4. Radioligand assay. QV126 N494]
QP364.7.N47 612'.8 78-3010
ISBN 0-89004-231-4

Preface

The use of ligand-binding techniques to study neurotransmitter receptor sites has led to a broad range of important biological advances. It is now possible to obtain information about the regional distribution of neurotransmitter receptors in brain, the pharmacological, biochemical, and developmental characteristics of these sites, and the functional interrelationships between neuronal cell types. In addition, the receptor-binding procedure has been used as an assay technique to measure levels of neurotransmitters and drugs, to identify new transmitter candidates, and to separate and purify receptors. The simplicity and versatility of these techniques render them attractive biochemical tools for routine use in neuroscience laboratories.

As with all methods, it is necessary to understand some of the basic principles of the technique in order to use a receptor-binding procedure appropriately. To this end, this text covers the fundamental principles of neurotransmitter receptor-binding assays, discusses the precise methodology for some of the more commonly used assays, and describes ways in which the assays can be used in neurobiological investigations, drug screening, neurochemical and histochemical analysis, and in the solubilization and isolation of receptors. This book is not intended as a review of the literature in these areas, but rather as a guide to enable neuroscientists, from technicians to senior investigators, to understand the basis of receptor-binding assays and to help establish these procedures in the laboratory. The utility and limitations of the binding assays in industrial drug screening, clinical medicine, and basic research are stressed.

Our chief goal has been to provide the reader with fundamental principles and procedures. Discussions of specific studies are limited to those that illustrate and clarify these principles. By using this approach, we hope that this book will serve not only as a laboratory guide but also as a catalyst for future investigations.

Henry I. Yamamura
S. J. Enna
Michael J. Kuhar

Acknowledgment

We would like to acknowledge our indebtedness to Solomon H. Snyder and to our other mentors: George Aghajanian, Akira Horita, Alfred Pletscher, Robert Roth, Lewis Schanker, and Parkhurst Shore.

Contents

Contributors

James P. Bennett, Jr.: *Department of Pharmacology, Johns Hopkins University School of Medicine, Baltimore, Maryland 21205*

David R. Burt: *Department of Pharmacology, University of Maryland School of Medicine, Baltimore, Maryland 21201*

Ian Creese: *Department of Pharmacology, Johns Hopkins University School of Medicine, Baltimore, Maryland 21205*

S. J. Enna: *Departments of Pharmacology and Neurobiology and Anatomy, University of Texas Medical School at Houston, P.O. Box 20708, Houston, Texas 77025*

Morley D. Hollenberg: *Division of Clinical Pharmacology, Departments of Medicine and Pharmacology, Johns Hopkins University School of Medicine, Baltimore, Maryland 21205*

Michael J. Kuhar: *Departments of Pharmacology and Psychiatry, Johns Hopkins University School of Medicine, Baltimore, Maryland 21205*

Jon M. Lindstrom: *Salk Institute, P.O. Box 1809, San Diego, California 92112*

Solomon H. Snyder: *Departments of Pharmacology and Psychiatry, Johns Hopkins University School of Medicine, Baltimore, Maryland 21205*

Henry I. Yamamura: *Department of Pharmacology, College of Medicine, University of Arizona Health Sciences Center, Tucson, Arizona 85724*

Neurotransmitter Receptor Binding, edited by
H. I. Yamamura et al.
Raven Press, New York © 1978.

1

Overview of Neurotransmitter Receptor Binding

Solomon H. Snyder

Departments of Pharmacology and Experimental Therapeutics, and Psychiatry and Behavioral Sciences, Johns Hopkins University School of Medicine, Baltimore, Maryland 21205

New areas of science often develop following the introduction of a novel technique. Such advances need not be particularly profound in terms of technological complexity. More frequently, the availability of new simple, sensitive, and specific procedures attracts the interest of large numbers of investigators with a resulting escalation in the rate of new findings. In psychopharmacology, the introduction during the mid-1950s of chemical assays for norepinephrine and serotonin that were sensitive, specific, and relatively simple sparked a vast body of research into the role of these substances in the brain and almost literally initiated the field of biochemical psychopharmacology. Relatively simple procedures for preparing fractions of brain tissue enriched in pinched-off nerve terminals or synaptosomes greatly accelerated the investigation of numerous chemicals as neurotransmitter candidates. The availability of radiolabeled biogenic amines and their precursors at high specific activity prompted investigations of transmitter uptake and turnover. Straightforward biochemical assays measuring tyrosine hydroxylase activity permitted the discovery of α-methyl-p-tyrosine and other agents as inhibitors of the enzyme, permitting analyses of catecholamine turnover and the regulation of tyrosine hydroxylase activity.

Neurotransmitter receptors may in most instances consist of at least two distinct components, the recognition or binding site and some second portion of the receptor which "translates" transmitter recognition into a second messenger, usually an alteration in ion permeability or accumulation of a cyclic nucleotide. The bulk of this book is devoted to the recognition site of neurotransmitter receptors, an area in which research has increased dramatically in recent years.

The notion that drugs and biologically active compounds act at specific receptor sites has been accepted since the turn of the century. In the case of neurotransmitters, much early evidence derived from neurophysiological investigations. Biochemical approaches to receptors lagged behind neurophysiological investigations and behind almost all biochemical research into synaptic events. By 1970 the biosynthesis, storage, release, and inactivation of numerous transmitters had been characterized biochemically while little was known of receptors at a biochemical level. Major problems involved specificity and sensitivity in assays detailed as follows. The most straightforward approach to identifying receptor sites would be to measure the binding of the radioactive transmitter or a related drug to membranes from an appropriate target organ. However, most transmitter candidates and drugs possess hydrophilic and hydrophobic portions which can interact by ionic as well as non-ionic means with numerous sites on biological membranes. The numbers of such nonspecific binding sites would be expected to exceed vastly the minute number of specific transmitter receptors. The problem of sensitivity arises for ligands with high receptor affinity. Unless radiolabeled forms of the ligand have a high enough specific activity to permit assay at concentrations as low or lower than the dissociation constant, the concentration of radioactive ligand which must be added to produce measurable radioactivity in the membranes may saturate specific receptors and label primarily nonspecific sites.

Paton and Rang (39) provided a pioneering paradigm for labeling neurotransmitter receptors in studies evaluating binding of ^{3}H-atropine to slices of guinea pig ileum. Although most of the binding involved nonspecific sites, a portion labeled muscarinic receptor sites. Because of the low specific activity of the ^{3}H-atropine employed, the receptor was not characterized in great detail and these elegant observations were not pursued on a large scale. Subsequently the reversible anticholinergic ^{3}H-quinuclidinyl benzilate has proved valuable for efficient labeling of muscarinic receptors with selectivity and low levels of nonspecific binding (60).

Rang and co-workers (16,19) subsequently employed muscarinic drugs with alkylating mustard properties as receptor labels. The shift from reversible to irreversible ligands by these workers reflects an ongoing debate between exponents of the two approaches. Alkylating agents may form potentially irreversible covalent links to receptor sites that can be valuable in attempts to monitor the receptor during solubilization and purification. However, the alkylated receptor usually lacks biological activity. Since the goal of solubilization and purification is to examine transmitter interactions with the receptor, alkylating the receptor may be akin to "cutting off your nose to spite your face." A potentially more serious problem relates to specificity. With reversible ligands receptors can be labeled selectively if the ligand has higher affinity for the receptor than for nonspecific binding sites. However, with incubations of sufficient duration an alkylating agent labels sites of low as well as of high affinity. One of the most successful uses of alkylating agents to label neurotransmitter receptors involves benzilyl choline mustards developed by Rang and co-workers (16,19) and subsequently by Burgen and his colleagues (5). The latter group utilized these mustards for autoradiographic visualization of the receptors, a task for which irreversible ligands are better suited than reversible ones.

Although historical priority may belong to studies of the muscarinic cholinergic receptor, the application of binding techniques to the nicotinic cholinergic receptor in 1970 attracted more scientific visibility and drew many scientists into the investigation of neurotransmitter receptors. A crucial ingredient in these studies was the ligand α-bungarotoxin. This polypeptide is a potent and almost irreversible antagonist at nicotinic cholinergic receptors. Using ^{125}I-labeled α-bungarotoxin, several workers (7,30,32,45) identified specific binding to nicotinic cholinergic receptor sites in membranes of the electric organ of the electric fish. α-Bungarotoxin was shown to have a dissociation constant in the nanomolar range and to dissociate only very slowly from binding sites. Nicotinic agonists and antagonists competed for binding with potencies which in general corresponded to their pharmacological activity whereas nonnicotinic agents lacked activity. Because α-bungarotoxin dissociated so slowly from receptor sites, it was possible to solubilize the nicotinic receptor with detergents such as Triton-X-100 and to purify the receptor extensively. In early studies it was shown that the bungarotoxin binding protein was a physically distinct entity from acetylcholinesterase, which refuted earlier hypotheses that these were both parts of the same macromolecule.

Even prior to the α-bungarotoxin investigations, O'Brien and associates had demonstrated binding interactions involving nicotinic cholinergic receptors in electric organs using ^{3}H-muscarone and assaying the binding by centrifugation (37) and equilibrium dialysis (38). The difficulty with equilibrium dialysis as a tool to detect binding interactions is that one measures a reduction in radioactivity of the ligand in the incubation medium so that small amounts of binding are not readily measured. Karlin and Cowburn (25) utilized unique nicotinic ligands which formed covalent associations with the receptor through sulfhydryl groups obtained after reduction of a disulfide bond of the receptor with dithiothreitol. Specificity was ensured by regarding as "specific" interactions only those which were prevented by omitting dithiothreitol.

Earlier studies of hormone receptors provided a major impetus to work with neurotransmitter receptor sites. The classic studies of Jensen and Jacobson (23) beginning in 1962 identified estradiol receptors. Jensen first demonstrated these receptors in intact animals by showing that target organs such as the uterus, vagina, and pituitary accumulated ^{3}H-estradiol in a saturable fashion which could be antagonized by steroids in proportion to their estrogen-like activity. A technical breakthrough making Jensen's studies feasible was his own synthesis of ^{3}H-estradiol of very high specific radioactivity. This was important because estrogen receptors have extremely high affinity for their hormone. Subsequently Jensen et al. (24), Gorski et al. (21), and other workers showed that estrogen and other steroid hormone receptors are cytoplasmic and move to the nucleus following interactions with their hormone. By contrast, neurotransmitter receptors are thought to be localized primarily to the external surface of neuronal membranes.

Receptors for peptide hormones historically have provided a more useful model for neurotransmitter receptors. Indeed it is now becoming evident that several peptide hormones may also serve neurotransmitter functions.

Studies of the insulin receptor by Cuatrecasas (11) and Roth and colleagues

(18) provided valuable information about receptor properties and technological approaches. In the case of peptides such as insulin, great care must be taken to ensure that labeling the hormone with ^{125}I does not impair biological activity. Overly rigorous iodination may add more than one iodine per insulin molecule, which interferes with biological and binding activity. Some studies of the insulin receptor have highlighted questions of specificity. For instance, it was shown that ^{125}I-insulin could bind with high affinity to talcum powder, and that the relative potencies of some insulin analogs in competing for binding paralleled their biological activity (12). Clearly numerous agents must be examined critically before concluding that the biologically meaningful receptor is being studied. In the case of insulin direct comparisons can be made between binding and physiological activity by measuring the oxidation of glucose as well as binding in intact fat cells. For central neurotransmitters the brain does not usually provide simple biochemical assays of physiological activity.

To detect specific receptor binding and to minimize nonspecific binding required technical innovations. In measuring insulin receptors Cuatrecasas assayed membrane-bound insulin by filtration with a manifold which permits the analysis of many samples simultaneously and an efficient vacuum which facilitates rapid but thorough washing to remove nonspecifically bound ligand without perturbing receptor-bound compound. These relatively simple technological principles have been of considerable importance for studies of central neurotransmitter receptors.

The logical sequence of events in neuropharmacology begins with a known neurotransmitter whose receptor interactions are characterized, and finally potential receptor-active drugs are evaluated. In the case of the opiate receptor this sequence was reversed. A historical description of efforts to characterize the opiate receptor illuminates some important methodological and theoretical issues. It had been well known that most pharmacological activities of opiates are stereospecific with the (−)-isomer possessing much greater potency than the (+)-isomer. Since the late 1950s numerous workers have attempted to measure the binding of radioactive opiates to brain membranes, using as their screen for selective interactions with the opiate receptor stereospecificity of displacement of binding by plus and minus isomers. In 1971 Goldstein et al. (20) noted that ^{3}H-levorphanol bound to membranes in mouse brain homogenates and that approximately 2% of the binding could be displaced stereospecifically by levorphanol but not by dextrorphan, the pharmacologically inactive isomer. The minute amount of stereospecific binding precluded detailed characterization. The specific activity of the ^{3}H-levorphanol employed was quite low so that high concentrations, approximately 0.1 mM, were added routinely. Because binding sites of high affinity would have been completely saturated at this concentrations, the binding sites evaluated by Goldstein et al. (20) would have had to possess relatively low affinity. Another puzzling aspect of these sites was their localization to nuclear fractions of brain homogenates and the fact that highest densities of the binding sites occurred in areas of the brain rich in white matter. Subsequently Goldstein succeeded in amplifying the amount of stereospecific binding and in solubilizing and purifying the binding substance. Loh et al. (29) then showed that the binding material did not contain protein but consisted almost exclusively of cerebrosides. Subsequently Abood and Hoss (1) showed that a variety of acidic lipids could bind opiates stereoselectively. Indeed even synthetic filters used in some binding studies bind radioactive opiates stereoselectively with the (−)-isomer being more potent than the (+)-isomer (51).

This story illustrates the importance of a detailed and rigorous demonstration of specificity of receptor interactions, preferably with comparisons of binding and biological activity in the same tissue. Thus the subsequent demonstration of high-affinity stereospecific binding of ^{3}H-opiates to brain membranes (41, 47,53) was a necessary but not sufficient criterion for identification of the opiate receptor. A correlation of binding potencies with analgesic activity provided further evidence. Most conclusive evidence derived from comparisons of binding affinities in membranes from the guinea pig ileum with pharmacological activities of opiate agonists and antagonists in the same tissue (8).

Besides providing lessons about technical approaches to receptor binding, the opiate receptor has afforded insights into the differences between agonist and antagonist interactions with neurotransmitter receptors and how recognition of the transmitter might be translated into changes in ion permeability. When assays were conducted with Tris buffers, agonists and antagonists did not differ in their affinities for binding sites (42). However, small concentrations of sodium markedly enhanced the binding of ^{3}H-opiate antagonists while diminishing the binding of ^{3}H-agonists (44). The effect of sodium was potent, occurring at 1 mM sodium, and selective, being manifested to a limited extent by lithium but not rubidium, cesium, or potassium (43). These findings were consistent with a model of the opiate receptor in which two interconvertible states prefer agonists and antagonists, respectively. The pharmacological properties of an antagonist occur because it binds to the "antagonist" state of the receptor, making fewer "agonist" states available for opiates or opioid transmitters. One can postulate that the ion whose permeability is relevant to transmission, in this case sodium, binds preferentially to one of the two states of the receptor, in this case the antagonist state. Normally receptor sites are bathed in sodium. By binding to the agonist state of the receptor, morphine would provoke a transformation of antagonist conformations of the receptor to agonist conformations, "loosening" the binding of sodium and thus altering its membrane permeability. A direct role of sodium has been demonstrated in mediating neurophysiological inhibitory influences of opiates and opioid peptides (63).

Interactions of the ion conductance modulator and receptor binding sites have also been apparent in studies of the glycine receptor. Glycine is thought to be a major inhibitory neurotransmitter in the spinal cord and lower brainstem. Glycine receptors can be labeled with the glycine antagonist ^{3}H-strychnine (61). Synaptic hyperpolarization elicited by glycine involves an increase in chloride conductance. Physiological concentrations of chloride reduce the binding of ^{3}H-strychnine and also decrease the affinity of glycine for the binding sites

(36,62). The ability of 14 anions to mimic this effect of chloride corresponds closely with their relative abilities to mimic the reversal of inhibitory postsynaptic potentials by chloride. Whether these binding interactions distinguish glycine agonists and antagonists has not been adequately investigated because it has not proved possible to label glycine receptors with glycine itself or another agonist.

Besides glycine, the other major inhibitory neurotransmitter in the brain is also an amino acid γ-aminobutyric acid (GABA). In contrast to the glycine receptor, which is best labeled with the antagonist strychnine, the GABA receptor has been most effectively studied by the binding of the agonist ^{3}H-GABA (64) or ^{3}H-muscimol (2,15). Recent studies of the GABA receptor with the antagonist ^{3}H-bicuculline (33) suggest that it may label a state of the receptor with preferential affinity for antagonists. However the apparent affinities of agonists and antagonists for sites of the GABA receptor labeled by ^{3}H-GABA and ^{3}H-bicuculline, respectively, do not differ as markedly as is the case for certain other receptors.

A prime candidate for the major excitatory transmitter in the brain is also an amino acid, glutamic acid. The evidence for glutamic acid as a transmitter is weaker than is the case for other amino acid transmitters, such as glycine or GABA. Kainic acid, a rigid analog of glutamic acid, is substantially more potent than glutamate in causing synaptic excitation. Binding sites labeled by ^{3}H-kainic acid exhibit a substrate specificity suggesting that the binding sites represent the physiological glutamate receptors (48).

Interactions between recognition and "second messenger" sites of a transmitter receptor have also been identified for β-noradrenergic receptors. In this case, the second messenger appears related to adenylate cyclase rather than to a specific ion. β-Receptors have been successfully labeled with ^{3}H-dihydroalprenolol (^{3}H-DHA), ^{3}H-propranolol, and ^{125}I-hydroxybenzylpindolol (^{125}I-HYP). Recently it has been possible to label β-receptors in some tissues with agonists such as ^{3}H-hydroxybenzylisoproterenol (28) and ^{3}H-epinephrine (55). Physiological desensitization of β-receptors by chronic exposure to catecholamines in frog erythrocytes is reflected in decreased responsiveness of the adenylate cyclase to stimulation by catecholamines. Desensitization is accompanied by a reduction in ^{3}H-DHA binding and a slowing of the dissociation of the agonist ^{3}H-hydroxybenzylisoproterenol associated with a higher affinity of the agonist (28,31,35). An increased affinity of transmitter for receptors had been postulated as the mechanism of desensitization at nicotinic receptors of the neuromuscular junction by Katz and Thesleff on physiological grounds (26). Enhanced agonist affinity at nicotinic receptors in preparation of electric organs during desensitization has also been demonstrated by Weber et al. (59). It is conceivable that such desensitization is a universal aspect of neurotransmitter receptor interactions. In any event, Mukherjee and Lefkowitz showed that guanyl nucleotides can reverse the physiological desensitization and simultaneously accelerate the dissociation of ^{3}H-hydroxybenzylisoproterenol from β-receptors (35). Under normal circumstances GTP and related nucleotides decrease the affinity of β-agonists for receptor sites but only in tissues that can be physiologically desensitized (e.g., frog but not turkey erythrocytes).

Distinct binding states for agonists and antagonists have been clearly demonstrated with dopamine and α-norepinephrine receptor in the brain. ^{3}H-Dopamine and ^{3}H-apomorphine appear to label agonist states of the dopamine receptor, whereas ^{3}H-haloperidol and ^{3}H-spiroperidol label antagonist preferring states (6,10,17,46). Thus dopamine agonists have substantially greater potency in competing for the binding of ^{3}H-dopamine than ^{3}H-haloperidol, and the reverse holds for dopamine antagonists. Agonist states of α-noradrenergic receptors can be labeled with ^{3}H-clonidine, ^{3}H-epinephrine, and ^{3}H-norepinephrine, and antagonist states can be labeled with ^{3}H-WB-4101, and ^{3}H-dihydroergokryptine behaves in an intermediate fashion (56–58). Whereas agonist and antagonist states of opiate and dopamine receptors appear to be interconvertible, the two binding states of the α-receptor are apparently distinct receptors. Although α-receptors are not traditionally thought to be associated with adenylate cyclase, influences of GTP and related nucleotides on α-receptor binding are essentially the same as on β-receptors in tissues in which desensitization can be demonstrated. Thus GTP diminishes the potencies of α-agonists and accelerates their dissociation from receptor sites.

Serotonin synaptic receptors can be labeled with the transmitter ^{3}H-serotonin (4). The binding of ^{3}H-LSD to brain membranes also has properties of serotonin receptors in most parts of the brain (3,4). Relative affinities of serotonin agonists, antagonists, and ergots suggest that ^{3}H-LSD behaves as a mixed agonist–antagonist in labeling serotonin receptors (4). In the corpus striatum, which is rich in dopamine neurons, approximately 20% of ^{3}H-LSD binding involves dopamine receptors while the majority remains associated with serotonin receptors. The possibility that a radioactive ligand can label a multiplicity of receptor sites is highlighted by studies of ^{3}H-dihydroergokryptine (^{3}H-DHE). In the rabbit uterus, ^{3}H-DHE binding appears exclusively associated with α-noradrenergic receptors (58). In the brain low concentrations of ^{3}H-DHE also selectively label α-receptors (22). However, at slightly higher concentrations (5 to 10 nM) ^{3}H-DHE labels serotonin as well as α-receptors in most brain regions (13), and in the corpus striatum ^{3}H-DHE labels dopamine receptors as well (54). Thus a single ligand can label three receptor sites in the brain. These findings are in accord with the pharmacological data that ergots such as DHE have potent effects at dopamine, α- and serotonin receptors.

Interestingly, the β-receptor does not seem to distinguish agonists and antagonists. Agonists and antagonists have similar potencies in competing for binding of agonists ^{3}H-hydroxybenzylisoproterenol and ^{3}H-epinephrine as in the binding of antagonists such as ^{3}H-DHA (27,28,56).

One of the most recent brain receptors to be identified is the benzodiazepine receptor (34,52). The relative potencies of benzodiazepines in competing for high-affinity binding of ^{3}H-diazepam closely parallels their pharmacological potencies. No other drugs or neurotransmitters examined have any substantial affinity for these binding sites. In analogy with the opiate receptor, it has been proposed that there may be some normally occurring benzodiazepine-like neurotransmitter.

Neurotransmitter receptor binding has led to a number of practical applications in industry as well as in research laboratories, some of which are detailed in later chapters of this book. Opiate and dopamine receptor binding assays are used routinely for screening potential analgesics and antischizophrenic drugs, respectively. Affinities of neuroleptics for muscarinic cholinergic (50) and α-noradrenergic receptors (40) predict extrapyramidal and sedative side effects of neuroleptics, respectively. The clinically important anticholinergic effects of tricyclic antidepressants and neuroleptics are predicted by their affinities for muscarinic cholinergic receptor binding (49).

Another practical application involves the use of receptor binding as a tool to measure drugs or neurotransmitters themselves. Such a radioreceptor assay for GABA (14) is at least as sensitive and specific as any other known assay and considerably simpler to perform. A radioreceptor assay for neuroleptic drugs has several virtues over other analytical procedures (9). Since the therapeutic effect of these drugs in schizophrenic patients derives from blockade of dopamine receptors, the assay can detect any of the large number of neuroleptic drugs marketed. Moreover, it monitors active metabolites as well as the parent drug.

In summary, in the course of a relatively few years studies of neurotransmitter receptors by binding techniques have made considerable advances. The most generally applicable approach to labeling receptors has been to utilize reversible ligands, either the transmitters themselves or appropriate agonist or antagonist drugs. Using these procedures receptor sites for almost all the known neurotransmitters in the peripheral and central nervous system can now be monitored biochemically. Binding assays have permitted an approach to relating recognition of the transmitter to some second messenger involving ion conductance changes or cyclic nucleotide alterations. Assays of neurotransmitter receptor binding have had practical ramifications in the design of new drugs and in radioreceptor assays.

REFERENCES

1. Abood, L. G., and Hoss, W. (1975): Stereospecific morphine adsorption to phosphatidyl serine and other membranous components of brain. *Eur. J. Pharmacol.,* 32:66–75.
2. Beaumont, K., Chilton, W., Yamamura, H. I., and Enna, S. J. (1978): Muscimol binding in rat brain: Association with synaptic GABA receptors. *Brain Res. (in press).*
3. Bennett, J. L., and Aghajanian, G. K. (1974): D-LSD binding to brain homogenates: Possible relationship to serotonin receptors. *Life Sci.,* 15:1935–1944.
4. Bennett, J. P., Jr., and Snyder, S. H. (1976): Serotonin receptor binding in rat brain membranes. *Mol. Pharmacol.,* 12:373–389.
5. Burgen, A. S. V., Hiley, C. R., and Young, J. M. (1974): The binding of ^{3}H-propylbenzilylcholine mustard by longitudinal muscle strips from guinea-pig small intestine. *Br. J. Pharmacol.,* 50:145–151.
6. Burt, D. R., Creese, I., and Snyder, S. H. (1976): Characteristics of ^{3}H-haloperidol and ^{3}H-

dopamine binding associated with dopamine receptors in calf brain membranes. *Mol. Pharmacol.,* 12:800–812.
7. Changeux, J-P., Kasai, M., Huchet, M., and Meunier, J-C. (1970): Extraction a partir du tissu electrique de gymnote d'une proteine presentant plusieurs proprietes characteristiques du recepteur physiologique de l'acetylcholine. *C. R. Acad. Sci. Paris,* 270:2864–2867.
8. Creese, I., and Snyder, S. H. (1975): Receptor binding and pharmacological activity of opiates in the guinea pig intestine. *J. Pharmacol. Exp. Ther.,* 194:205–219.
9. Creese, I., and Snyder, S. H. (1977): A simple and sensitive radioreceptor assay for antischizophrenic drugs in blood. *Nature (Lond.),* 270:180–182.
10. Creese, I., Schneider, R., and Snyder, S. H. (1977): ^{3}H-Spiroperidol labels dopamine receptors in pituitary and brain. *Eur. J. Pharmacol.,* 46:377–381.
11. Cuatrecasas, P. (1971): Insulin-receptor interaction in adipose tissue cells: Direct measurement and properties. *Proc. Natl. Acad. Sci. USA,* 68:1264–1268.
12. Cuatrecasas, P., and Hollenberg, M. D. (1975): Binding of insulin and other hormones to non-receptor materials: Saturability, specificity and apparent "negative cooperativity." *Biochem. Biophys. Res. Commun.,* 62:31–41.
13. Davis, J. N., Strittmatter, W., Hoyler, E., and Lefkowitz, R. J. (1977): ^{3}H-Dihydroergokryptine binding in rat brain. *Brain Res.,* 132:327–336.
14. Enna, S. J., and Snyder, S. H. (1976): A simple, sensitive and specific radioreceptor assay for endogenous GABA in brain tissue. *J. Neurochem.,* 26:221–224.
15. Enna, S. J., Beaumont, K., and Yamamura, H. I. (1978): Comparison of ^{3}H-muscimol and ^{3}H-GABA receptor binding in rat brain. In: *Amino Acids as Chemical Transmitters,* edited by F. Fonnum. Plenum Press, New York *(in press).*
16. Fewtrell, C., and Rang, H. P. (1971): Distribution of bound ^{3}H-benzilylcholine mustard in subcellular fractions of smooth muscle from guinea pig ileum. *Br. J. Pharmacol.,* 43:417P.
17. Fields, J. Z., Reisine, T. D., and Yamamura, H. I. (1977): Biochemical demonstration of dopaminergic receptors in rat and human brain using ^{3}H-spiroperidol. *Brain Res.,* 136:578–584.
18. Freychet, P., Roth, J., and Neville, D. M., Jr. (1971): Insulin receptor in the liver: Specific binding of ^{125}I-insulin to the plasma membrane and its relation to insulin bioactivity. *Proc. Natl. Acad. Sci. USA,* 68:1833–1837.
19. Gill, E. W., and Rang, H. P. (1966): An alkylating relative to benzilylcholine with specific and long-lasting parasympatholytic activity. *Mol. Pharmacol.,* 2:284–297.
20. Goldstein, A., Lowney, L. I., and Pal, B. K. (1971): Stereospecific and nonspecific interactions of the morphine congener levorphanol in subcellular fractions of the mouse brain. *Proc. Natl. Acad. Sci. USA,* 68:1742–1747.
21. Gorski, J., Taft, D., Shyomala, G., Smith, D., and Notides, A. (1968): Hormone receptors: Studies on the interaction of estrogen with the uterus. *Recent Prog. Horm. Res.,* 24:45–80.
22. Greenberg, D. A., and Snyder, S. H. (1977): Selective labeling of α-noradrenergic receptors in rat brain with ^{3}H-dihydroergokryptine. *Life Sci.,* 20:927–932.
23. Jensen, E. V., and Jacobson, H. I. (1962): Basic guides to the mechanism of estrogen action. *Recent Prog. Horm. Res.,* 18:387–414.
24. Jensen, E. V., Suzuki, T., Kawashima, T., Stumpf, W. E., Jungblut, P. W., and DeSombre, E. R. (1968): A two-step mechanism for the interaction of estradiol with rat uterus. *Proc. Natl. Acad. Sci. USA,* 59:632–638.
25. Karlin, A., and Cowburn, D. A. (1973): The affinity-labeling of partially purified acetylcholine receptor from electric tissue of Electrophorus. *Proc. Natl. Acad. Sci. USA,* 70:3636–3640.
26. Katz, B., and Thesleff, S. (1957): A study of the 'desensitization' produced by acetylcholine at the motor end-plate. *J. Physiol. (Lond.),* 138:63–80.
27. Lefkowitz, R. J., and Hamp, M. (1977): Comparison of specificity of agonist and antagonist radioligand binding to β-adrenergic receptors. *Nature (Lond.),* 268:453–455.
28. Lefkowitz, R. J., and Williams, L. T. (1977): Catecholamine binding to the β-adrenergic receptor. *Proc. Natl. Acad. Sci. USA,* 74:515–519.
29. Loh, H. H., Cho, T. M., Wu, Y-C., and Way, E. L. (1974): Stereospecific binding of narcotics to brain cerebrosides. *Life Sci.,* 14:2231–2245.
30. Meunier, J-C., Olsen, R. W., Menez, A., Fromageot, P., Boquet, P., and Changeux, J-P. (1972): Some physical properties of the cholinergic receptor protein from Electrophorus electricus revealed by a tritiated α-toxin from Naja nigricollis venom. *Biochemistry,* 11:1200–1210.
31. Mickey, J., Tate, R., and Lefkowitz, R. J. (1975): Subsensitivity of adenylate cyclase and

decreased β-adrenergic receptor binding after chronic exposure to (−)-isoproterenol in vitro. *J. Biol. Chem.*, 250:5727–5729.
32. Miledi, R., Molinoff, P., and Potter, L. T. (1971): Isolation of the cholinergic receptor protein of Torpedo electric tissue. *Nature (Lond.)*, 229:554–557.
33. Mohler, H., and Okada, T. (1977): GABA receptor binding with ^{3}H-bicuculline methiodide in rat CNS. *Nature (Lond.)*, 267:65–67.
34. Mohler, H., and Okada, T. (1977): Benzodiazepine receptor: Demonstration in the central nervous system. *Science*, 198:849–851.
35. Mukherjee, C., and Lefkowitz, R. J. (1976): Desensitization of β-adrenergic receptors by β-adrenergic agonists in a cell-free system: Resensitization by guanosine-5′-(β,γ-imino)triphosphate and other purine nucleotides. *Proc. Natl. Acad. Sci. USA*, 73:1494–1498.
36. Muller, W. E., and Snyder, S. H. (1978): Strychnine binding associated with synaptic glycine receptors in rat spinal cord membranes: Ionic influences. *Brain Res. (in press)*.
37. O'Brien, R. D., and Gilmour, L. P. (1969): A muscarone-binding material in electroplax and its relation to the acetylcholine receptor. I. Centrifugal assay. *Proc. Natl. Acad. Sci. USA*, 63:496–503.
38. O'Brien, R. D., Thompson, W. R., and Gibson, R. E. (1974): A comparison of acetylcholine and α-bungarotoxin binding to soluble Torpedo receptor. In: *Neurochemistry of Cholinergic Receptors*, edited by E. de Robertis and J. Schact, pp. 49–62. Raven Press, New York.
39. Paton, W. D. M., and Rang, H. P. (1965): The uptake of atropine and related drugs by intestinal smooth muscle of the guinea-pig in relation to acetylcholine receptors. *Proc. Roy. Soc. B*, 163: 1–44.
40. Peroutka, S. J., U'Prichard, D. C., Greenberg, D. A., and Snyder, S. H. (1977): Neuroleptic drug interactions with norepinephrine alpha-receptor binding sites in rat brain. *Neuropharmacology*, 16:549–556.
41. Pert, C. B., and Snyder, S. H. (1973): Opiate receptor: Demonstration in nervous tissue. *Science*, 179:1011–1014.
42. Pert, C. B., and Snyder, S. H. (1973): Properties of opiate-receptor binding in rat brain. *Proc. Natl. Acad. Sci. USA*, 70:2243–2247.
43. Pert, C. B., and Snyder, S. H. (1974): Opiate receptor binding of agonists and antagonists affected differentially by sodium. *Mol. Pharmacol.*, 10:868–879.
44. Pert, C. B., Pasternak, G., and Snyder, S. H. (1973): Opiate agonists and antagonists discriminated by receptor binding in brain. *Science*, 182:1359–1361.
45. Raftery, M. A., Schmidt, J., Clark, D. G., and Wolcott, R. G. (1971): Demonstration of a specific α-bungarotoxin binding component in Electrophorus electricus electroplax membranes. *Biochem. Biophys. Res. Commun.*, 45:1622–1629.
46. Seeman, P., Chau-Wong, M., Tedesco, J., and Wong, K. (1975): Brain receptors for antipsychotic drugs and dopamine: Direct binding assays. *Proc. Natl. Acad. Sci. USA*, 72:4376–4380.
47. Simon, E. J., Hiller, J. M., and Edelman, I. (1973): Stereospecific binding of the potent narcotic analgesic ^{3}H-etorphine to rat brain homogenate. *Proc. Natl. Acad. Sci. USA*, 70:1947–1949.
48. Simon, J. R., and Kuhar, M. J. (1976): Specific ^{3}H-kainic acid binding to rat brain membranes: Evidence for association with the L-glutamate receptor. *J. Neurochem.*, 141–147.
49. Snyder, S. H., and Yamamura, H. I. (1977): Antidepressants and the muscarinic acetylcholine receptor. *Arch. Gen. Psychiatry*, 34:236–239.
50. Snyder, S. H., Greenberg, D., and Yamamura, H. I. (1974): Antischizophrenic drugs and the brain cholinergic receptors. *Arch. Gen. Psychiatry*, 31:58–61.
51. Snyder, S. H., Pasternak, G. W., and Pert, C. B. (1975): Opiate receptor mechanisms. In: *Handbook of Psychopharmacology*, Vol. 5, edited by L. L. Iversen, S. D. Iversen, and S. H. Snyder, pp. 329–360. Plenum Press, New York.
52. Squires, R. F., and Braestrup, C. (1977): Benzodiazepine receptors in rat brain. *Nature (Lond.)*, 266:732–734.
53. Terenius, L. (1973): Characteristics of the "receptor" for narcotic analgesics in synaptic plasma membrane fraction from rat brain. *Acta Pharmacol. Toxicol.*, 33:377–384.
54. Tittler, M., Weinreich, P., and Seeman, P. (1977): New detection of brain dopamine receptors with [^{3}H]dihydroergocryptine. *Proc. Natl. Acad. Sci. USA*, 74:3750–3753.
55. U'Prichard, D. C., and Snyder, S. H. (1977): Differential labelling of α- and β-noradrenergic receptors in calf cerebellum membranes with ^{3}H-adrenaline. *Nature (Lond.)*, 270:261–263.
56. U'Prichard, D. C., and Snyder, S. H. (1977): Binding of ^{3}H-catecholamines to α-noradrenergic receptor sites in calf brain. *J. Biol. Chem.*, 252:6450–6463.

57. U'Prichard, D. C., Greenberg, D. A., and Snyder, S. H. (1977): Binding characteristics of a radiolabeled agonist and antagonist at central nervous system alpha noradrenergic receptors. *Mol. Pharmacol.,* 13:454–473.
58. Williams, L. T., Mullikin, D., and Lefkowitz, R. J. (1976): Identification of α-adrenergic receptors in uterine smooth muscle membranes by ^{3}H-dihydroergokryptine binding. *J. Biol. Chem.,* 251:6915–6923.
59. Weber, M., David-Pfeuty, T., and Changeux, J-P. (1975): Regulation of binding properties of the nicotinic receptor protein by cholinergic ligands in membrane fragments from Torpedo marmorata. *Proc. Natl. Acad. Sci. USA,* 72:3443–3447.
60. Yamamura, H. I., and Snyder, S. H. (1974): Muscarinic cholinergic binding in rat brain. *Proc. Natl. Acad. Sci. USA,* 71:1725–1729.
61. Young, A. B., and Snyder, S. H. (1973): Strychnine binding associated with glycine receptor in the central nervous system. *Proc. Natl. Acad. Sci. USA,* 70:2832–2836.
62. Young, A. B., and Snyder, S. H. (1974): The glycine synaptic receptor: Evidence that strychnine binding is associated with the ionic conductance mechanism. *Proc. Natl. Acad. Sci. USA,* 71:4002–4005.
63. Zieglgansberger, W., and Bayerl, H. (1976): The mechanism of inhibition of neuronal activity by opiate in the spinal cord of cat. *Brain Res.,* 115:111–128.
64. Zukin, S. R., Young, A. B., and Snyder, S. H. (1974): Gamma-aminobutyric acid binding to receptor sites in the rat central nervous system. *Proc. Natl. Acad. Sci. USA,* 71:4802–4807.

Neurotransmitter Receptor Binding, edited by
H. I. Yamamura et al.
Raven Press, New York © 1978.

2

Receptor Models and the Action of Neurotransmitters and Hormones

Morley D. Hollenberg

Division of Clinical Pharmacology, Departments of Medicine and Pharmacology, Johns Hopkins University School of Medicine, Baltimore, Maryland 21205

I. INTRODUCTION

The study of the binding of a variety of neurotransmitter molecules and drugs to putative pharmacological receptors is entering an exciting phase. As detailed elsewhere in this volume and in a number of recent review articles (7,21,31,34,44), sufficient expertise has now been developed to measure with confidence the interaction of radioactive ligand probes with infinitesimally small numbers of high-affinity binding sites in cell or membrane preparations. In most cases the measurement of ligand binding, when placed in the context of the criteria outlined in Chapter 3 and developed elsewhere (31), can be shown to be characteristic of "true" pharmacological receptors. Such studies have now led to the accumulation of an enormous amount of data (summarized in refs. 6–8,21,26,29,31,36,44) concerning these receptors, comprising information such as their molecular weights, the kinetics of receptor turnover (23), the phosphorylation of receptor substituents (28,49), and their localization at the cellular and subcellular level. The challenge at the present time is to integrate the empirical information obtained into a mechanistic construct that will explain in detail the manner whereby ligand recognition is translated into an integrated cellular and tissue response.

The concept of the receptor is inextricably linked to the biological responsiveness of a system (enzyme, cell, or tissue) to a neurotransmitter or hormone of particular interest. Indeed, prior to 1965 practically all of the information concerning receptors was deduced from an analysis of dose–response data for a variety of agonist and antagonist compounds, with a great deal of that work focused primarily on neurotransmitter agents causing rapid effects in nerve/muscle preparations. From the analysis of the responsiveness of such systems (e.g., ion flux, force of contraction, rate of contraction), a number of theoretical models of drug action have been proposed. It is important to note that the derivation and presentation of some of the models are clearly biased in terms of neurotransmitter action (e.g., opening and closing of ion channels) such that the models, although in many respects general, may not be applicable to the action of certain compounds such as steroids that act via intracellular receptors rather than via plasma membrane receptors.

It is the object of this chapter to focus on a number of receptor models that have been proposed for drugs or hormones that are thought to initiate a biological response via interactions with receptors located in the plasma membrane. No attempt is made either to present each model in complete detail or to present a comprehensive review of all models of drug action that have been described, since comprehensive derivations and reviews are already readily available (e.g., 2,6,8,16,26,33,35). Rather, an overview is presented of a number of models of drug action that have been and should continue to be of value in planning an experimental approach to the problem of neurotransmitter action. Ultimately, the various models proposed will have to accommodate observations of the kind described elsewhere in this volume.

II. DOSE–RESPONSE CURVES AND THE RELATION BETWEEN LIGAND BINDING AND BIOLOGICAL RESPONSE

A. General Considerations

It is a fundamental assumption of any receptor theory, as stated explicitly by Ehrlich, that for an agent to act it must be bound. The site of initial recognition and binding, termed the "receptor," can thus, to a first approximation, be thought of in relatively simple chemical terms according to a bimolecular neurotransmitter–receptor interaction.[1]

$$R + H \underset{k_{-1}}{\overset{k_1}{\rightleftharpoons}} RH \rightarrow \rightarrow \text{Response} \qquad [1]$$

Where H = hormone or neurotransmitter, R = receptor, RH is the receptor–hormone complex, and the equilibrium dissociation constant, K_D, is given by the quotient of the rate constants, k_{-1}/k_1. This simple equilibrium forms the basis for a number of theories of drug action that focus either on the equilibrium concentration of receptor–hormone complex ("occupancy assumption") as developed by Clark (13–16), Gaddum (24,25), Ariens (1,2), Stephenson and co-workers (46,47), and others, or on the rates of formation and dissociation of the receptor–hormone complex, as emphasized by the "rate theory" developed by Paton and co-workers (39–41). It is to be noted that Clark as well (16) fully appreciated the mechanistic implications of the rates of drug action. Although as outlined below, the "rate theory" and "occupancy theories" differ with regard to the immediate function of the hormone receptor complex, both theories regard the complex as a distinct physicochemical entity with properties different from those of the uncomplexed components. Thus as further details concerning the sequence of biochemical events leading to cellular activation by neurotransmitters become available, the differences between the "rate" and "occupancy" theories may appear somewhat arbitrary; that is, on the one hand, the rates of interaction must become a consideration for "occupancy theories," and, on the other hand, the biochemical mechanisms concerning the occupied, "inert" drug receptor complex must be dealt with by the "rate" theories.

B. Equations Based on the "Occupancy" Assumption

It is a tenet of the occupancy theories that the magnitude of the biological response is in some way proportional to the amount of ligand–receptor complex formed [RH]. If a bimolecular reaction is assumed, as given by Eq. [1], at equilibrium, according to the law of mass action, the dissociation constant K_D of the ligand–receptor complex is given by

$$K_D = ([H][R])/[RH] \qquad [2]$$

where [H], [R], and [RH] represent the concentrations of *free* hormone, receptor, and receptor–hormone complex, respectively. In its simplest form, as developed by Clark (13–16) and Gaddum (24,25), the occupancy theory assumes that there is a direct proportionality between the concentration of receptor–hormone complex [RH] and the pharmacological effect, Q, which may be expressed

$$Q = \alpha[RH] \qquad [3]$$

[1] In this chapter the terms "neurotransmitter," "drug," and "hormone" are used interchangeably to represent the ligands with which receptors interact.

where α is a proportionality constant. Further, it is assumed that there is no response elicited by unoccupied receptors and that the maximum response, Q_{max}, is attained when all receptors are occupied; that is,

$$Q_{max} = \alpha[R_T] \qquad [4]$$

where $[R_T]$ is the total receptor concentration, given by the sum of free and complexed receptor

$$[R_T] = [R] + [RH] \qquad [5]$$

substituting Eq. [5] into Eq. [2] and rearranging

$$[RH]/[R_T] = [H]/(K_D + [H]) \qquad [6]$$

Since

$$Q/Q_{max} = [RH]/[R_T]$$

it follows that

$$Q = Q_{max}[H]/(K_D + [H]) \qquad [7]$$

Eq. [7], derived on the basis of the initial assumptions, indicates a hyperbolic relationship between the response and the *free* concentration of hormone; the concentration of hormone producing a half-maximal response $[H]_{0.5}$ (usually termed the ED_{50}) can be equated with the equilibrium dissociation constant for the hormone–receptor interaction.

The form of Eq. [7] is identical to that of the well-known substrate–velocity relationship of enzyme kinetics; in Eq. [7], Q_{max} represents the more familiar V_{max} and Q replaces V, the reaction velocity. It is thus possible to use all of the mathematical relationships of enzyme kinetics developed for enzyme substrates (drug agonists) and enzyme inhibitors (drug antagonists). It is important to point out, however, that as far as has been determined, hormones are not metabolized by receptors as are enzyme substrates by specific enzymes. In addition to the assumption of proportionality between occupancy and response as indicated by Eqs. [3] and [4], Eq. [7] presupposes a simple bimolecular reaction between hormone and receptor. In practice, dose–response curves usually depict response versus a function of $[H_T]$, the total concentration of drug present in the assay system, on the assumption that the proportion of bound drug is very small, such that $[H_T] \simeq [H]$, the free drug concentration. Should an appreciable fraction of drug be bound, then the total concentration of hormone $[H_T]$, at which response is 50% of maximum, will exceed the K_D by an amount equal to one-half of the total concentration of receptor, as indicated in the following derivation:

If f represents the fraction of the maximum response ($0 < f \leq 1$) at a given hormone concentration,

$$f = Q/Q_{max} = [RH]/[R_T] \qquad [8]$$

then from Eq. [6]

$$f = [\mathrm{H}]/(K_D + [\mathrm{H}]) \qquad [9]$$

which by rearranging gives

$$[\mathrm{H}] = K_D[(f)/(1-f)] \qquad [10]$$

since $[\mathrm{H_T}] = [\mathrm{H}] + [\mathrm{RH}]$, and from Eq. [8], $[\mathrm{RH}] = f[\mathrm{R_T}]$, one can substitute into Eq. [10] to obtain

$$[\mathrm{H_T}] = K_D[f/(1-f)] + f[\mathrm{R_T}] \qquad [11]$$

It thus appears that under certain experimental conditions receptor concentration can become an important consideration for the analysis of dose–response data, just as enzyme concentration may prove to be a factor in the analysis of substrate–velocity relationships, as emphasized by Straus and Goldstein (48). When $[\mathrm{R_T}]$ is very small (i.e., the concentration of bound drug, $f[\mathrm{R_T}]$ is negligible), then

$$[\mathrm{H_T}] = K_D[f/(1-f)] \qquad [11a]$$

and at the half-maximal response, $f = 0.5$, $[\mathrm{H_T}]_{0.5} = K_D$. When $\mathrm{R_T}$ becomes very large with respect to the K_D, then in the extreme

$$[\mathrm{H_T}] = f[\mathrm{R_T}] \qquad [11b]$$

such that a linear relationship between total drug concentration and fractional response may obtain. From Eq. [11] it is seen, as indicated above, that the total concentration of ligand at which response is half-maximal is given by

$$[\mathrm{H_T}]_{0.5} = K_D + 0.5[\mathrm{R_T}] \qquad [11c]$$

The same considerations concerning receptor concentrations apply to the analysis of ligand-binding data (Chapter 4), as dealt with in detail by Rodbard (42).

For many pharmacological studies with nerve and muscle preparations and with isolated cells such as adipocytes, the concentration of receptors is indeed well below the estimated K_D of the receptor–ligand interaction. For instance, insulin-mediated enhancement of glucose transport in adipocytes is half-maximal at a concentration of approximately 3×10^{-11} M insulin. From the available experimental data (approximately 2×10^5 cells/ml used in an assay, with 10^4 receptors per cell) (18), the receptor concentration can be estimated to be 3×10^{-12} M. The $[\mathrm{H_T}]_{0.5}$ or $\mathrm{ED_{50}}$ for insulin action might thus be taken as a theoretical estimate of the receptor K_D for insulin, based on bioassay measurements, neglecting the last term of Eq. [11] and assuming a linear occupancy–response relationship, i.e., Eqs. [3] and [4] are assumed to be true.

The data in Fig. 1 illustrate some of the considerations discussed above. The solid lines represent theoretical curves based on Eq. [11] (curves a to f) for different concentrations $[\mathrm{R_T}]$ of a receptor possessing a hypothetical ligand dissociation constant of 5×10^{-11} M. Curve a represents Eq. [11a]; curve f approximates Eq. [11b]. The right hand ordinate, f, can be taken to represent

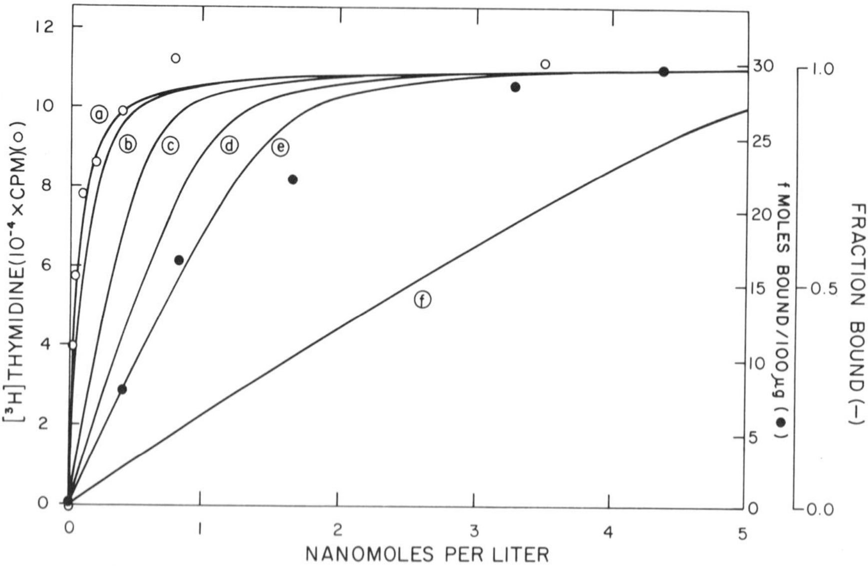

FIG. 1. Biological response and epidermal growth factor (EGF) binding in human fibroblast monolayers. Plots of total hormone concentration ($[H_T]$, in nanomoles/liter) versus fractional binding (equivalent to fractional response by Eq. [11]; solid lines, right ordinate) were generated by computer using Eq. [11] assuming an equilibrium dissociation constant of 5×10^{-11} M and various concentrations of receptor: $[R_T]$ for curve a = 0; b = 10^{-10} M; c = 5×10^{-10} M; e = 1.5×10^{-9} M; f = 5×10^{-9} M. Experimental data for measurements of EGF binding (●) and the biological response to EGF (thymidine incorporation) (○) are superimposed on the theoretical curves. (From Cuatrecasas and Hollenberg, ref. 21.)

either fractional binding of a ligand to a receptor or the fractional biological response. The difficulty in interpreting an ED_{50} without knowledge of either the *free* concentration of hormone or of the total concentration of receptor $[R_T]$ is apparent in Fig. 1.

Superimposed on the theoretical curves (a to f) in Fig. 1 are dose–response (○) and receptor-binding (●) data obtained in identical human fibroblast monolayers (i.e., R_T is the same for both measurements) for the polypeptide epidermal growth factor–urogastrone (EGF/URO; see refs. 9,30,32). A receptor concentration of approximately 3×10^{-11} M can be estimated in such experiments; this value is almost an order of magnitude smaller than the estimated K_D for EGF/URO binding. The experimental data in Fig. 1 are illustrative of the noncoincidence of dose–response curves (○) and hormone-binding curves (●) for the same cells. This noncoincidence can be observed not only for EGF/URO but also for other agonist compounds in a variety of cell systems. This situation can be contrasted with the coincidence of the dose–response curve and hormone binding isotherm that can be measured for insulin action in isolated adipocytes (18).

C. Simple Occupancy Assumptions and the Interpretation of Dose–Response Data

The discordance between the ED_{50} for a biological response and the K_D estimated by the binding of agonists may prove to be the rule rather than the exception, as illustrated by the following relatively simple derivations. It is evident that the more removed the ultimate biological response is from the initial ligand interaction, the more complicated the "coupling" between receptor occupation and cellular activation might be, even within the framework of a straightforward occupancy model. The introduction of a single constant term into Eq. [3] demonstrates several complications. If response, Q, is related to receptor occupation by the equation

$$Q = a[\mathrm{RH}] + A \qquad [12]$$

where the constant A can be allowed negative values and where the proportionality constant a may differ from the one (α) previously described, then the maximum response, when all receptors are occupied, may be written in analogy with Eq. [4]:

$$Q_{\max} = a[\mathrm{R_T}] + A \qquad [13]$$

Two simple situations can be depicted: (a) where the signal generated by the hormone–receptor complex is sufficient for a maximal response with only a certain fraction of receptors, p, occupied (a "spare" receptor situation, to be discussed below), where

$$Q_{\max} = a(p[\mathrm{R_T}]) + A \qquad [14]$$

or (b) where a certain threshold signal must be generated by occupancy of a minimal fraction, S, of the available receptors; that is, $S = [\mathrm{R_{min}}]/[\mathrm{R_T}]$, before a response is observable. At "threshold" receptor occupancy, where there still is no response ($Q = 0$), $[\mathrm{RH}] = [\mathrm{R_{min}}] = S[\mathrm{R_T}]$, and from Eq. [12]: $A = -aS[\mathrm{R_T}]$. Three possibilities are considered:

1. $S = 0$; $0 < p \leq 1$ (fractional receptor occupancy gives a maximum response) p is the fraction of receptors occupied when response is maximal.
2. $0 < S \leq 1$; $p = 1$ (a threshold receptor occupancy is required for response) S is the minimum fraction of receptors occupied to give an observable response.
3. $0 < S \leq 1$; $0 < p < 1$ where for a response to occur, p must be greater than S. [A combination of situations (1) and (2)].

For situation (1), since $Q = 0$ when $[\mathrm{RH}] = 0$, from Eq. [12], $A = 0$ (i.e., $Q = a[\mathrm{RH}]$). Since the maximum response is achieved at fractional receptor occupancy (i.e., $Q_{\max} = ap[\mathrm{R_T}]$), in analogy with Eq. [8], fractional response may be expressed

$$Q/Q_{\max} = [\mathrm{RH}]/p[\mathrm{R_T}] = f \qquad [15]$$

From Eq. [6], substituting for $[RH]/[R_T]$,

$$fp = [H]/(K_D - [H]) \quad [16]$$

Since the total receptor concentration is the sum of that which is free and that which is bound to receptor (i.e., $[H_T] = [H] + [HR]$), substituting from Eq. [15], $[H] = [H_T] - fp[R_T]$. Now substituting for [H] in Eq. [16] and rearranging

$$[H_T] = K_D[fp/(1 - fp)] + fp[R_T] \quad [17]$$

which is identical in form to Eq. [11]. When $[R_T]$ is small with respect to K_D, the right hand term of Eq. [17] can be neglected and the 50% response (ED_{50}; $f = 0.5$) in terms of total hormone concentration for such a response ($[H_T]_{0.5}$) is given by the equation

$$[H_T]_{0.5} = [p/(2 - p)]K_D \quad [18]$$

By plotting the ratio $[H_T]_{0.5}/K_D$ versus p as indicated in Fig. 2, it is evident that in all cases where more receptors are present than the number required

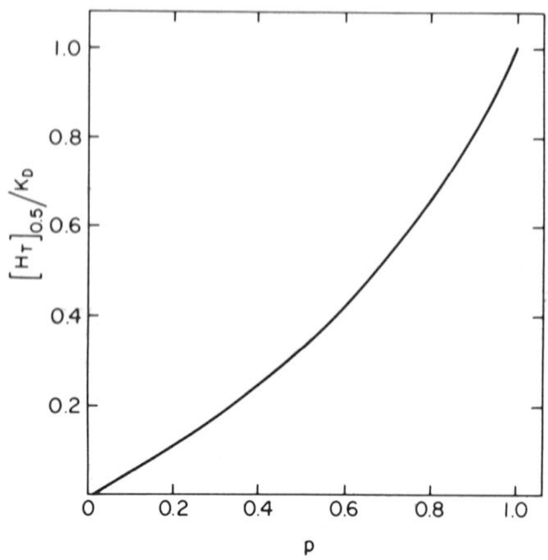

FIG. 2. Theoretical occupancy–response relationship. Relationship between $[H_T]_{0.5}/K_D$ and the fraction p, of receptors occupied for a maximal response. (From Cuatrecasas and Hollenberg, ref. 21.)

for a maximal response (spare receptors) $[H_T]_{0.5}/K_D$ will always be less than unity and the ED_{50} will *underestimate* the value of the true K_D.

When a "threshold" phenomenon obtains [situation (2)], as mentioned above, $A = -aS[R_T]$, and from Eqs. [12] and [13], $Q = a[RH] - aS[R_T]$; $Q_{max} = a[R_T] - aS[R_T]$. Thus

$$\frac{Q}{Q_{max}} = f = \frac{[RH] - S[R_T]}{[R_T]\ (1 - S)} \quad [19]$$

and therefore

$$[RH]/[R_T] = f(1 - S) + S \quad [20]$$

Again, substituting in Eq. [6] for $[RH]/[R_T]$ and noting that $[H] = [H_T] - [RH]$, and that $[RH] = [R_T][f(1 - S) + S]$, one obtains

$$[H_T] = \frac{K_D[f(1 - S) + S]}{1 - [f(1 - S) + S]} + [f(1 - S) + S][R_T] \qquad [21]$$

again, assuming $[R_T]$ is negligible, one obtains from Eq. [21] that when response is half-maximal ($f = 0.5$),

$$[H_T]_{0.5}/K_D = (1 + S)/(1 - S) \qquad [22]$$

The plot of $[H_T]_{0.5}/K_D$ versus S as determined by Eq. [22] and illustrated in Fig. 3 demonstrates that where a "threshold" receptor occupancy is required to provide an observable biological response, the ED_{50} (or $[H_T]_{0.5}$) will always *overestimate* the value of the true K_D.

It can be derived similarly for case 3, where a fractional threshold occupancy, S, is necessary to initiate a response, and a maximal response is attained with a fractional occupancy, p, that

$$[H_T] = \frac{K_D[f(p - S) + S]}{1 - [f(p - S) + S]} + [f(p - S) + S][R_T] \qquad [23]$$

For low receptor concentrations and $f = 0.5$, the equation becomes

$$[H_T]_{0.5}/K_D = (p + S)/[2 - (p + S)] \qquad [24]$$

the plot of $[H_T]_{0.5}/K_D$ versus $(p + S)$ as determined from Eq. [24] is shown in Fig. 4.

It can be seen that only in the case where $(p + S)$ is unity can the value of $[H_T]_{0.5}$ equal the K_D. It can be appreciated that for a drug to act, S and p cannot both be unity. Additionally the quantity $(p - S)$ can be seen to represent the "working range" of the receptor, as indicated schematically in Fig. 5. Similarly, the fraction $(1 - p)$ represents the proportion of receptors not needed to

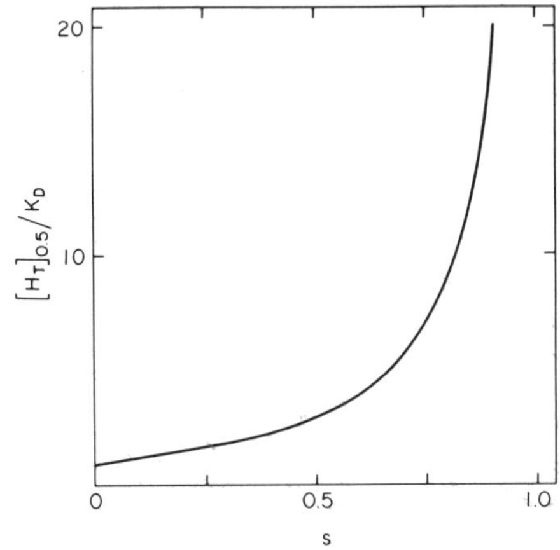

FIG. 3. Theoretical occupancy–response relationship. Relationship between $[H_T]_{0.5}/K_D$ and the fraction, S, of receptors that must be occupied for a threshold response. The ordinate intercept starts at 1.0, when $S = 0$. (From Cuatrecasas and Hollenberg, ref. 21.)

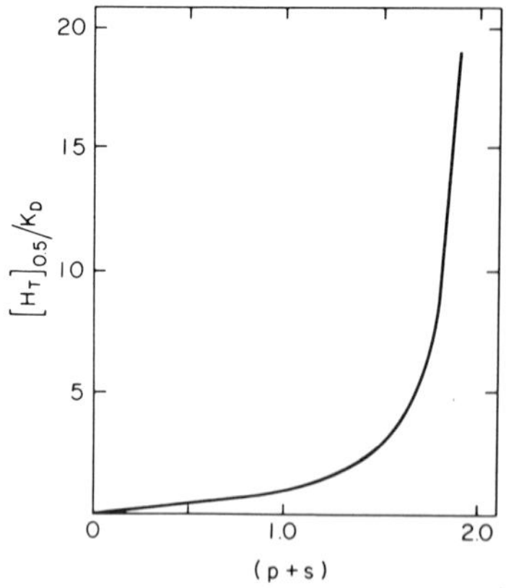

FIG. 4. Theoretical occupancy–response relationship. Relationship between $[H_T]_{0.5}/K_D$ and receptor occupancy *(p + S),* where a threshold response is not observed until the fraction, *S,* of receptor is occupied, and where a maximum response is observed with a fraction, *p,* occupied. (From Cuatrecasas and Hollenberg, ref. 21.)

generate a given response ("spare" receptors). It can be seen that as the magnitude of *S* approaches that of *p* (and, by definition, *S,* must always be less than *p* for a response to occur) the "working range" of the receptor becomes narrower, so as to approach the situation where an "all or none" response may occur for a receptor that can exhibit a normal binding isotherm. In such a case it may be difficult if not impossible to estimate an $[H_T]_{0.5}$ from the biological dose–response data and another approach is necessary (e.g., see ref. 47). It is one of the goals of ligand-binding studies to estimate the magnitude of *S* and *p,* as depicted schematically in Fig. 5.

From the above derivations, based on relatively simple and somewhat naive assumptions concerning receptor occupation and tissue activation, it should be evident as to how difficult it is to deduce from dose–response curves the quantitative characteristics of the initial hormone–receptor interaction. Any biological estimate of the affinity of an agonist for its receptor requires an assumption as to the coupling of hormone binding to a biological response. The complexity of events between hormone binding and response in most systems (e.g., measurement of muscle contraction) thus precludes a detailed analysis of concentration–

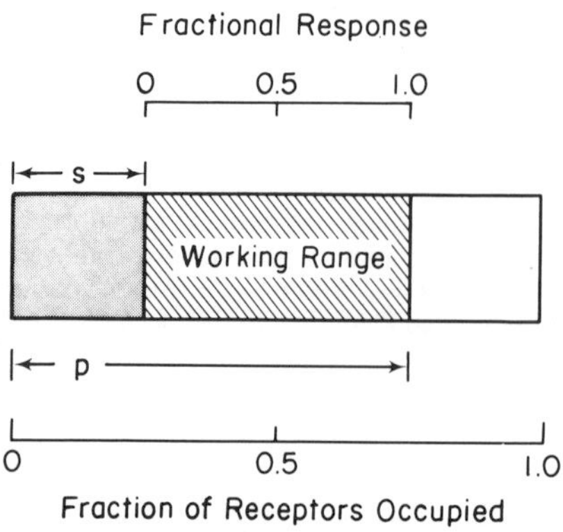

FIG. 5. Schematic representation of receptor occupation. A hypothetical situation is depicted where a threshold effect is observed and where "spare" receptors are present. A response is not measurable until a fraction, *S,* of receptors is occupied and a maximum response is generated by occupation of a fraction, *p,* of receptors. (From Cuatrecasas and Hollenberg, ref. 21.)

effect curves. Detailed analyses (discussed below) have nonetheless been developed for neurotransmitter–receptor interactions where response, measured in terms of ionic conductance, is thought to reflect directly the number of ion channels opened by a drug.

Despite the above reservations, it is important to note that data from many pharmacological experiments are consistent with Eq. [11a]. In order to represent responsiveness over a wide range of concentrations, fractional response is usually plotted as a function of log [H_T] so as to yield a sigmoid curve with an inflection point at the $ED_{50}(f = 0.5)$; the theoretical value of the slope of the curve at this point is 0.576 (for derivation, see ref. 27). In situations where trivial complications, such as ligand degradation, variability due to different methods of recording responsiveness, or potentiation of responsiveness by nonreceptor factors [e.g., presence of an inhibitor of cyclic adenosine monophosphate (cAMP) phosphodiesterase in a system responding to the level of cAMP] can be ruled out, the $[H_T]_{0.5}$ or ED_{50} from dose–response curves can be used as a reasonable first approximation of the affinity of the hormone–receptor interaction. Furthermore, the relative ED_{50}'s for agonists yielding parallel dose–response curves with the same maximum response (e.g., curves a and b, Fig. 6) can be taken as representative of the relative affinity of agonists for the receptor. Most importantly, the

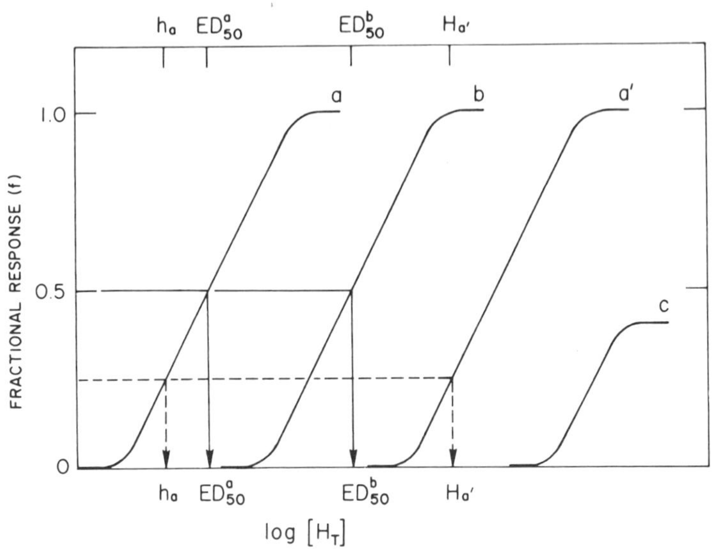

FIG. 6. Schematic dose-response curves. The plots of fractional response *(f)* versus total hormone concentration (log [H_T]) are shown. Curves a and b (with different ED_{50} values) represent the action of two drugs in a congeneric series, acting at the same receptor site with different affinities; curve c represents the action of a partial agonist in such a series. Curve a′ represents the action of drug a in the presence of a competitive antagonist; h_a and $H_{a'}$ represent the concentration of drug a necessary to yield the same response in the absence and presence of the competitive antagonist (see Eqs. [28] and [29]).

dose–response data provide the essential foundation for the interpretation of ligand-binding data, as described elsewhere in this volume, where it is important to be able to distinguish receptor binding from nonreceptor binding artifacts.

D. Competitive Antagonists

Although it is true, as discussed above, that information concerning the receptor–agonist equilibrium constant cannot be deduced from concentration–effect curves, this is not the case for drug antagonists. The basis for the estimate of antagonist affinities by bioassay as developed by Schild and co-workers (3,45) is derived below. In the derivation of the relationships for antagonists, a simple, truly competitive, bimolecular interaction between either agonist or antagonist and receptor is assumed. Furthermore, the derivation rests on the principle of the "null" hypothesis, whereby it is assumed that when the response to one concentration of agonist, h, in the absence of inhibitor, A, is the same as the response to a higher concentration of agonist, H, in the presence of competitive inhibitor, then the amount of agonist reaching the receptor in the two situations is identical (compare curves a and a′, Fig. 6). The equilibria can be written

$$\mathrm{R} + \mathrm{H} \rightleftarrows \mathrm{RH}, \text{ RH is pharmacologically active} \qquad [25]$$

$$\mathrm{R} + \mathrm{A} \rightleftarrows \mathrm{RA}, \text{ RA is inactive} \qquad [25a]$$

Let y represent, for a given response, the proportion of receptors occupied: $y = [\mathrm{RH}]/[\mathrm{R_T}]$, where, as above, [RH] represents the concentration of hormone–receptor complex and $[\mathrm{R_T}]$ the total concentration of receptor present. If, for a given response, [H] represents the free concentration of hormone when antagonist is present, with [A] = free concentration of antagonist, K_A = equilibrium association constant for the antagonist, and K_H = equilibrium association constant for the hormone, then, in the presence of a hormone antagonist it can be derived from the mass action equation corresponding to Eqs. [25] and [25a] that

$$K_\mathrm{H}[\mathrm{H}] = \{(1 + [\mathrm{A}]K_\mathrm{A})\}\, y/(1 - y) \qquad [26]$$

If the *same* biological response is observed in the *absence* of antagonist (i.e., A = 0 and y, the proportion of receptors occupied remains unchanged), at a lower concentration of the hormone, [h], then

$$K_\mathrm{H}[\mathrm{h}] = y/(1 - y) \qquad [27]$$

Dividing Eq. [26] by Eq. [27]

$$[\mathrm{H}]/[\mathrm{h}] = 1 + [\mathrm{A}]K_\mathrm{A} \qquad [28]$$

Eq. [28] represents the so-called Schild equation, wherein [H]/[h] is the "dose ratio," as depicted in Fig. 6 by the ratio of the values Ha′/*h*a.

Theoretically, the dose ratio is constant (curves a and a′ in Fig. 6 are parallel) regardless of the response level chosen. This prediction has held true in a number of studies of different drugs over a wide range of concentrations.

For the concentration of antagonist, $[A]_2$, where the hormone concentration must be doubled to achieve the same effect observed without antagonist (i.e., $[H]/[h] = 2$), one obtains from Eq. [28]

$$[A]_2 = 1/K_A \tag{28a}$$

The equilibrium association constant of the antagonist can therefore be determined by bioassay, without any assumption as to the relationship between the proportion of receptors occupied and the size of the response, since the magnitude of the response is kept constant. It should be pointed out that the concentrations [A], [H], and [h] shown in Eq. [28] represent the *free* concentrations of the ligands. In practice, biological measurements are done without a knowledge of the amount of ligand complexed; it is assumed that the total concentrations of ligands $[H_T]$, $[h_T]$, and $[A_T]$ approximate the actual free concentrations. For systems of very high affinity, where an appreciable concentration of receptor may be present, such may not be the case. Thus, if the proportion of receptor occupied by hormone, H, is $y = [RH]/[R_T]$, and that occupied by antagonist, A, is $z = [RA]/[R_T]$, Eq. [28] can be rewritten in terms of *total* ligand concentrations for the situation where the same response is observed, with the total concentration of ligands given by

$$[H_T] = [H] + [RH] = [H] + y[R_T]$$

$$[h_T] = [h] + [Rh] = [h] + y[R_T]$$

$$[A_T] = [A] + [RA] = [A] + z[R_T]$$

Thus, substituting in Eq. [28]

$$\frac{[H_T] - y[R_T]}{[h_T] - y[R_T]} = 1 + K_A([A_T] - z[R_T]) \tag{29}$$

When $[A_T]$ is such that $[H_T] = 2[h_T]$, then

$$[A_T]_2 = \frac{[h_T]}{K_A([h_T] - y[R_T])} + z[R_T] \tag{30}$$

It can be seen that for measurements at low-receptor occupancy (for both hormone and antagonist) and at low-receptor concentrations, Eq. [30] reduces to Eq. [28a]. It is assumed that no degradation of either hormone or antagonist occurs, and that simple bimolecular ligand–receptor interactions are involved. As pointed out by Chang and co-workers (10), the above equations apply equally to either the analysis of dose–response data or to the analysis of ligand-binding data, where a labeled ligand probe represents the "agonist," the unlabeled compound represents the competitive antagonist, and fractional receptor occupancy by labeled ligand represents fractional "response," as depicted in Fig. 6.

Alternatively, the interaction of either the radioactively labeled ligand or the unlabeled parent compound can be thought of in terms of the interaction of either a substrate or an inhibitor with an enzyme of interest. All of the equations of enzyme kinetics derived for the analysis of inhibitor (antagonist) action can be used directly for the interpretation of receptor–ligand interaction.[2] The radioactively labeled ligand can be thought of as the enzyme substrate (thus the specific ligand binding measured because the counterpart of "velocity"), and the parent unlabeled compound that competes for the binding of the labeled ligand can be taken to represent the "inhibitor" or antagonist of the reaction (i.e., the inhibitor reduces the "reaction velocity," or binding in a concentration-dependent manner). Thus, from a Dixon-type analysis of the binding of labeled ligand (substrate) in the presence of increasing concentrations of unlabeled ligand (inhibitor), an inhibitor affinity constant, K_i, can be determined: the plot of inhibitor concentration (unlabeled ligand) on the abscissa versus 1/reaction velocity (i.e., 1/binding of labeled ligand) on the ordinate is done for two or more fixed concentrations of substrate (i.e., labeled ligand). The intersection point of the family of straight lines so generated corresponds on the x-axis to the negative value of the K_i. This approach has been used successfully to estimate the receptor affinity of unlabeled mouse and human EGF/URO in cultured human fibroblast monolayers (31). In practice, binding–inhibitor data are frequently determined for only a single concentration of labeled ligand, and the concentration of unlabeled ligand that reduces the binding of labeled ligand by 50% (frequently termed the IC_{50}) is used to compute the "inhibitor" K_i from the formula

$$K_i = IC_{50}/\left(1 + \frac{L^*}{K^*}\right) \quad [31]$$

where K^* is the dissociation constant of the labeled ligand and L^* is the concentration of labeled ligand. Only where $K^* \gg L^*$ can the IC_{50} be taken to represent the K_i. Use of the above method to obtain the K_i yields the value for the *unlabeled* ligand. Again it is important to mention that, in the usual derivation of the equations for enzyme inhibitor, the concentration of enzyme is equally neglected, as is the case for the derivation of Eq. [31]. As discussed elsewhere (10,48), the concentration of receptor (or enzyme) may become an important factor, should the receptor concentration exceed one-tenth the value of the ligand dissociation constant. From the foregoing discussion it should be apparent that thinking of receptors and their ligands in terms of the mathematical formalism already well developed for enzymes and enzyme inhibitors (see Chapter 4 for an expanded discussion) can be useful in the interpretation of the kind of binding data discussed elsewhere in this volume.

---

[2] For derivation of the approximate formulae, the reader is referred to any modern text dealing with enzyme kinetics.

III. ALTERNATIVES TO THE SIMPLE OCCUPANCY THEORY

A. Phenomena Unaccounted for by the Simple Occupancy Theory

A number of interesting phenomena are observed in connection with the effects of hormones that must ultimately be explained by any proposed mechanism of agonist action: (a) Some antagonists, such as nicotine, first stimulate and then block a particular response. (b) Some compounds in a congeneric series of agonists do not elicit a full biological response, while at the same time blocking the action of more potent agents. Such compounds are called "partial agonists." (c) The concentration–effect curves for certain responses, such as membrane depolarization, do not follow a simple hyperbolic curve as predicted by Eqs. [7] or [11a]. (d) Repetitive exposure of a responsive tissue to an agonist for a prolonged time or at a high concentration of agonist leads to a diminished or absent sensitivity to the same compound (so-called "tachyphylaxis" if receptor-specific or desensitization if receptor nonspecific). (e) As alluded to above, either a full biological response may be elicited when only a fraction of the available receptors are occupied (i.e., "spare" receptors are present) or a response may not be generated until a certain proportion of receptors are occupied (a threshold effect). The above observations have led to the proposal of alternatives to the simple occupancy theory.

B. Rate Theory

From studies of histamine-mediated desensitization in smooth muscle and from a study of the kinetics of action of certain agonists (histamine and acetylcholine) and antagonists (hyoscine and mepyramine), Paton (39) was led to suggest that the effect produced by a drug depends not on the *number* of receptors occupied, but on the *rate* of receptor occupation by a drug.

Instead of attributing excitation to the occupation of receptor by drug molecules, Paton attributes excitation to the *process* of receptor occupation, each association between a drug molecule and a receptor providing one quantum of excitation. The process of occupation was envisioned in terms of an ion exchange at the receptor involving potassium and the active drug.

In this theory, Eq. [9] is written in terms of the association (k_1) and dissociation (k_{-1}) rate constants, whereby at equilibrium, fractional receptor occupancy, f, (fractional response, in terms of classical occupancy theory) is given by

$$f = [\mathrm{H}]/\{(k_{-1}/k_1) + [\mathrm{H}]\} \qquad [32]$$

and A, the rate at which drug combines with receptor (which rate at equilibrium equals the rate of drug dissociation from receptors $k_{-1}f$), will be given by

$$A = k_1[\mathrm{H}](1 - f) = k_{-1}f \qquad [33]$$

Substituting for f from Eq. [32] into [33]

$$A = \frac{k_{-1}[\mathrm{H}]}{[\mathrm{H}] + k_{-1}/k_1} \qquad [34]$$

The rate theory as developed by Paton and co-workers (39–41) proposes that Q, the equilibrium tissue response, is proportional to A, the rate of hormone-receptor complex formation; that is, $Q = \Phi\ A$, where Φ is the factor relating the intensity of chemical stimulation to tissue response. When nearly all of the receptors are occupied (f approaches 1), Eq. [33] gives $A = k_{-1}$. The rate theory predicts that the maximal response is directly proportional to the dissociation rate constant: slowly dissociating compounds will give small or negligible maximal responses (i.e., antagonists are predicted to have slower off-rates than are agonists).

The rate theory neatly accounts for the stimulatory action of antagonists and for drug-specific fading of an initial response, but less satisfactorily outlines suitable mechanisms at the molecular level. Furthermore, although concerns about diffusion barriers were rejected in the derivation of the rate theory, subsequent work (50) indicates that the rate of access of a drug to the receptor region is an important consideration. Importantly, the derivation of the rate theory provided a means of estimating by bioassay the association and dissociation rate constants so as to determine receptor affinities from the kinetic constants. The values thereby obtained for drug antagonists were in excellent agreement with equilibrium bioassay measurements (dose ratio), and a remarkably good agreement between both bioassay measurements and the equilibrium dissociation constant measured by ligand binding was observed for atropine by Paton and Rang (40). It is to the credit of the development of the rate theory that close attention is now given to the on-and-off-rates of ligand–receptor interactions and to the possibility that receptors once occupied by agonists may have to be recycled in some manner during the process of cellular activation. The advantages and shortcomings of this theory have been extensively discussed by Waud (51).

C. Intrinsic Activity or Drug Efficacy and "Spare Receptors"

Faced with the observations that some drugs, such as certain congeners of acetylcholine, do not cause a maximum biological response even at very high concentrations (e.g., curve c, Fig. 6), Ariens (1,2), Stephenson (46,47), and their co-workers were led to modify the simple occupancy theory discussed above. For the first time, two aspects of drug–receptor interactions were considered separately in a formal manner: (a) the recognition and binding of a ligand by the receptor (ligand affinity) and (b) the perturbation of the receptor to elicit a biological response (ligand "intrinsic activity," according to Ariens, or "efficacy," according to Stephenson). In essence, the proportionality constant of Eq. [3] is factored into a drug-specific constant (α or e) and a general proportionality constant, *a,* relating the intensity of the chemical stimulation to biological response.[3] Eq. [3] is then rewritten

$$Q = \Theta\,[RH] \qquad [35]$$

where

$$\Theta = \text{either } \alpha a \text{ (Ariens)} \quad \text{or } ea \text{ (Stephenson)}$$

In terms of the above construct, drugs can be classified in terms of two constants, α (or e), and the equilibrium dissociation constant, K_D. According to Ariens' theory, α will be zero for antagonists and unity for full agonists, an intermediate value for α will obtain for compounds classified as "partial agonists." In the derivations by Stephenson, the possibility is included that not all receptors need be occupied to elicit a full biological response (spare receptors). Additionally, it is considered that certain drugs may need to activate fewer of the available receptors to elicit a full biological response (i.e., some drugs are more "efficacious" than others). Thus the α of Ariens, which does not distinguish between drugs with $\alpha = 1$, is not equivalent to the e of Stephenson.

The concept of "spare" receptors embodied in the approach of Stephenson requires some amplification. Given that one is concerned with truly *equivalent* ligand-binding sites on a cell, it is important to realize that the same initial ligand receptor interaction may generate a signal (e.g., elevated levels of cAMP) that result in more than one cellular response. Thus given that different responses may require different levels of cAMP, the number of "spare" receptors observed may differ substantially, depending on the final response monitored. The concept becomes further complicated by a consideration of the cellular "effector" with which a hormone–receptor complex may interact to generate a cellular response (see discussion of the mobile receptor hypothesis below). Variations in the ratio of receptor to effector under certain circumstances may markedly alter the number of "spare" receptors determined by bioassay. In terms of overall cellular function, none of the available receptors for endogenous hormones may go unused.

In mechanistic terms, the efficacy or intrinsic activity of drugs might be thought of in terms of the ability of compounds to act as allosteric modulators of enzyme activity, that is, the receptor conformation. According to this paradigm, full agonists ($\alpha = 1$) might be envisioned as being able to cause a maximal shift in the K_m of the receptor for an endogenous substrate, present at a fixed concentration, so as to generate a reaction velocity sufficient for a maximal response; partial agonists might only be able to cause a partial shift in the

---

[3] In this context, the constants α and a take on a different significance than is defined for these symbols previously in Eqs. [3], [12], etc. The symbols are retained, in view of their use elsewhere in the literature in connection with the derivations of Ariens, Stephenson, and co-workers.

receptor "K_m." Increased drug "efficacy" may be thought of in terms of changing not only the receptor K_m but also the maximum turnover number; that is, less receptor would have to be in the "low K_m" state to generate the same reaction velocity for a fixed level of endogenous substrate. The above arguments are in keeping with a "macromolecular perturbation theory" of drug action developed by Belleau (4). Alternative considerations dealing with agonist-mediated changes in the receptor have led to an "induced-fit" model, in connection with the studies of the binding and biological action of muscarinic cholinergic agonists (6). In the "induced-fit" model, it is proposed that the active and inactive forms of the receptor possess different affinities for the agonist and that the ratio of agonist affinities relates to drug efficacy (6).

D. Multi-State Models and the Mobile Receptor Paradigm of Hormone Action

1. Two-State Models

The observation of sigmoid concentration–effect curves for agents such as carbachol and γ-aminobutyric acid that could not be attributed to artifacts of measuring the response (ionic conductance) led to the development of cooperative models for drug action. The sigmoid curves, in contrast to the hyperbolic concentration–effect curves depicted in Fig. 1, clearly resembled either the sigmoid oxygen-binding curves observed for hemoglobin or the sigmoid velocity–substrate relationship observed for certain enzymes. The model of Monod et al. (38) concerning the nature of allosteric transitions has therefore been adapted to models of drug action. Based on electrophysiological data, it was concluded that the membrane component(s) involved in ion transport (ion "channels") are thought to exist in two states, either open or shut, irrespective of the drug responsible for the modulation of conductivity. In the cooperative receptor models, it is assumed that the hormone receptor and ionophore form a strongly interacting membrane-localized complex (the drug-binding "protomer") that can exist in only two conformations for which the affinity of drug molecules may be different. The situation is depicted in Fig. 7, where in the absence of any ligand, the protomer will adopt an equilibrium between the T (closed) and R (open) states defined by the constant $K_L = [T]/[R]$. In the presence of either hormone or antagonist, the equilibrium between the T and R states of the protomer(s) is perturbed, depending on the values of the overall equilibrium dissociation constants of the ligands for the two protomer states, as depicted in Fig. 7.

In the case of potent agonists, it is proposed that the affinity of the hormone for the R state is much greater than that for the T state; that is, $K_{HR} \ll K_{HT}$. Agonists will therefore shift the equilibrium to the R state and open channels. In contrast, for antagonist compounds, it is supposed that the ligand affinity for the T state is much greater than that for the R state; that is, $K_{IT} \ll K_{IR}$, as depicted in Fig. 7. The equilibrium in the presence of antagonist would

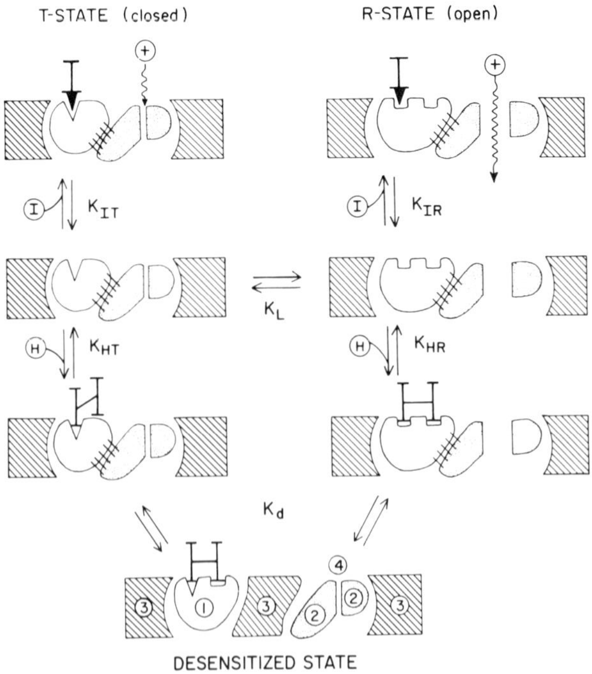

FIG. 7. Two-state model for hormone action. The receptor protomer is postulated to exist in either a T (ion channel closed) or R (ion channel open) state, with differential affinities for either a hormone, H, or inhibitor, I, determined by the equilibrium constants K_{IR}, K_{HR}, K_{IT}, K_{HT}. The proportion of receptors in the T or R states determines membrane conductivity. In the "desensitized" situation, determined by the overall equilibrium constant, K_d, the ligand recognition site (1) is separated from the ionophore (2) by other membrane constituents (3) and the ion channel (4) is closed. Differences in ligand-recognition site affinities are portrayed by different "lock and key" configurations. The strong association between the receptor and the ion channel is depicted by the oblique (hatched) lines.

thus favor the closed T state, providing for the possibility that antagonists could "close" pores that, depending on the value of K_L, might be open in the absence of any ligands. Because of the supposed preferential affinity of agonists for the R state and antagonists for the T state, the two states of the receptor protomers have also been referred to as agonist (R) and antagonist (T) state. The possibility is also depicted in Fig. 7 that, under certain conditions, the receptor protomer might be dissociated into a recognition moiety uncoupled from the ionophore. In such a "desensitized" situation, the recognition subunit(s) might be expected to possess ligand affinities distinct from those of either the T or the R state. The observation of high- and low-affinity sites for the binding of muscarinic agonists (6) may be rationalized in terms of the two-state model.

Two basic variations of the two-state model have been developed, as outlined extensively by Colquhoun (17), and in detail by Karlin (35), and by Changeux and co-workers (11,12). The "independent subunit" model supposes that there need be no cooperativity between ligand-binding sites, but that in order for membrane channels to open, a certain number, n, of protomers as depicted in Fig. 7 must be associated in the R conformation. The equilibria for a single protomer in the presence of hormone, H, are given by

$$\begin{array}{ccc} \mathrm{H+T} & \overset{K_L}{\rightleftharpoons} & \mathrm{R+H} \\ K_{HT}\upharpoonleft\downharpoonright & & \upharpoonleft\downharpoonright K_{HR} \\ \mathrm{HT} & & \mathrm{HR} \end{array}$$

If, for example, four protomers must associate in the R state to open a pore, then a sigmoid concentration–effect curve will result, with a Hill coefficient (see Chapter 4 for a discussion of the Hill equation) greater than unity (17).

Alternatively, it may be supposed that n protomers, instead of being independent, are all linked in some way, such that all n are constrained to adopt the same conformation; there are still only two membrane states, R_n (open) or T_n (shut). The equilibria in the presence of hormone, H, are given by

$$\begin{array}{ccc} \mathrm{nH+T_n} & \overset{K_L}{\rightleftharpoons} & \mathrm{R_n+nH} \\ K_{TH}\upharpoonleft\downharpoonright & & \upharpoonleft\downharpoonright K_{RH} \\ \mathrm{T_nH} & & \mathrm{R_nH} \\ K_{TH}\upharpoonleft\downharpoonright & & \upharpoonleft\downharpoonright K_{RH} \\ \mathrm{T_nH_n} & & \mathrm{R_nH_n} \end{array}$$

where K_L represents the equilibrium constant $[T_n]/[R_n]$ for the "concerted" transition between the two states and K_{RH} and K_{TH} represent the microscopic equilibrium dissociation constants for the interaction of the hormone with binding sites in the R and T states. This model (also termed the Monod–Wyman–Changeux or MWC model) also predicts sigmoid concentration–effect curves with Hill coefficients greater than unity. A comparison of the above cooperative models with the classic models for drug action has been discussed at length by Colquhoun (17).

The above cooperative theories not only rationalize on a mechanistic basis the complicated concentration effect curves measured electrophysiologically, but also provide a framework in which to evaluate complicated ligand-binding data. Clearly these models predict that a single membrane-localized receptor recognition macromolecule can be expected to display more than one affinity for a given ligand. Additionally, a "desensitized" state of the recognition molecule can be envisioned to have binding properties distinct from those of the ionophore-associated macromolecule. A disadvantage of the above theories is the sharply biased interpretation in terms of ionophores and ion pores. The mobile receptor model, to be described below, can be seen as a more generalized version of the two-state models.

2. The Mobile Receptor Model

Whereas the two-state models outlined above imply a restricted association between an ionophore and the ligand recognition sites, the "mobile" or "floating" receptor model developed simultaneously by Cuatrecasas and colleagues (5,19–21,33) and by DeHaën (22), proposes that a hormone–receptor complex may interact with a number of "effector" substituents in the plane of the membrane, as depicted in Fig. 8. The genesis for the theory centers around the observation that a number of receptor-specific agonists (catecholamines, prostaglandins, glucagon, ACTH, etc.) can independently stimulate adenylate cyclase in a cell such as the adipocyte in a manner indicative of a unique adenylate cyclase enzyme responding in a complex way to various hormonal stimuli. Rather than supposing that all of the receptors are clustered about the cyclase enzyme complex (this very large complex, which would be readily visible at the electron microscope level, has not been observed), it is proposed that each independent hormone–receptor moiety can freely compete for the effector (adenyl cyclase) in the plane of the membrane. The model, as depicted in Fig. 8, does not restrict the number of effectors with which the hormone–receptor complex may interact (e.g., an ion transport channel may be perturbed as well as a membrane enzyme complex) and the model is generally applicable to the modulation of any membrane process by a variety of hormones.

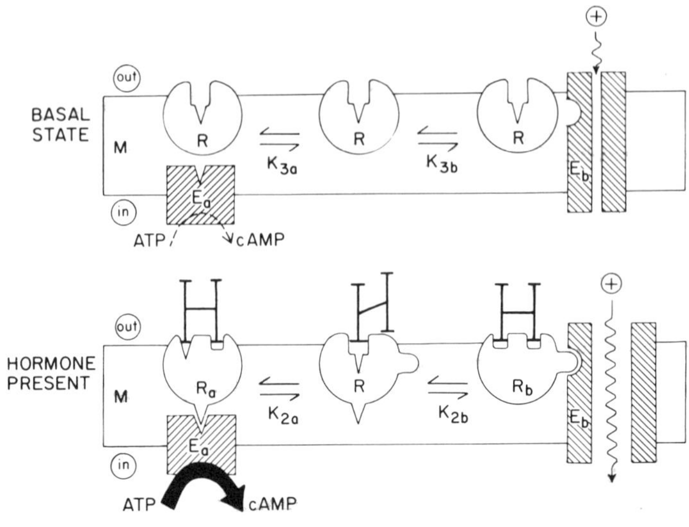

FIG. 8. Mobile receptor model of hormone action. The ability of the hormone-receptor complex to interact in the plane of the membrane is shown for two effector macromolecules: E_a = adenylate cyclase, converting adenosine 5′-triphosphate to adenosine 3′,5′-cyclic monophosphate (cAMP). E_b = transport system for a monovalent cation (depicted as a closed or open membrane pore). The equilibria are portrayed schematically in terms of the equilibrium constants expressed by Eqs. [36] and [37] in the absence **(top)** and presence **(bottom)** of a hormone agonist, H. The differences in hormone affinities between the uncomplexed and complexed states (receptor conformations R_a and R_b) are indicated by different "lock and key" configurations; the possible (weak) association between receptor and effectors in the absence of hormone is also shown. Only the ternary complex (HRE) is fully active, either converting ATP to cyclic AMP at an accelerated rate (HR_aE_a) or opening an ion channel (HR_bE_b). A receptor site for the binding of an inhibitor, like that depicted in Fig. 7, to form a nonassociating complex (IR; not shown) is also depicted. (out) Outside of cell; (in) inside of cell; (M) Cell membrane.

In a simplified version, the equilibria involved in the mobile receptor model can be expressed

$$\mathrm{mH} + \mathrm{R_m} \underset{k_{-1}}{\overset{k_1}{\rightleftharpoons}} \mathrm{R_mH_m} \qquad K_1 = \frac{k_1}{k_{-1}} \tag{36}$$

$$\mathrm{n(R_mH_m)} + \mathrm{E_n} \underset{k_{-2}}{\overset{k_2}{\rightleftharpoons}} \mathrm{E_n(R_mH_m)n} \qquad K_2 = \frac{k_2}{k_{-2}} \tag{37}$$

where H, R, and E represent hormone, receptor, and effector (e.g., membrane-bound adenyl cyclase), respectively, and where m and n are integers that may account for either multiple hormone-binding sites on the receptor or multimeric receptor species, as well as a complex interaction between the hormone–receptor complex and the effector. It is evident that the equilibria could readily be made more complex, so as to account for cooperative phenomena, by varying the stoichiometry of the reacting species (e.g., either the receptors or effector may well represent oligomeric macromolecular species), as represented by the integers m and n. Indeed, should receptors exist as clusters within the plane of the membrane, negative cooperativity between receptor molecules alone could account for "spare" receptors as discussed by Levitzki (37), whereby low ligand occupancy would lead to a large configural change of the receptor cluster. The values, K_1 and K_2 represent the microscopic equilibrium association constants for the reactions with overall forward and reverse rate constants, k_1, k_{-1}, k_2, and k_{-2}. In the simplest case, both m and n will be unity. It is a fundamental hypothesis of the mobile receptor model that the affinity of the hormone–receptor complex for the effector, as expressed by the equilibrium constant, K_2, is greater than the affinity of the uncomplexed receptor for the effector, as given by the following equation:

$$\mathrm{nR_m} + \mathrm{E_n} \underset{k_{-3}}{\overset{k_3}{\rightleftharpoons}} \mathrm{E_n(R_m)_n} \qquad K_3 = \frac{k_3}{k_{-3}} \tag{38}$$

and expressed by the equilibrium constant K_3. It is thus proposed that for a hormone inhibitor, I, it would be expected that the ternary complex (IRE) (depicted as HRE in Fig. 8) would be biologically inactive and that for the inhibitor, K_2 would equal K_3. A fourth equilibrium that can occur is the dissociation of the hormone–receptor–effector complex according to the equation

$$(\mathrm{m} \cdot \mathrm{n})\mathrm{H} + \mathrm{(R_m)_nE_n} \underset{k_{-4}}{\overset{k_4}{\rightleftharpoons}} \mathrm{(H_mR_m)_nE_n} \qquad K_4 = \frac{k_4}{k_{-4}} \tag{39}$$

An even more generalized scheme than the one described by the above four equations has been described by De Haën (22) for the action of hormones that stimulate adenylate cyclase.

If it is assumed that $\mathrm{m} = \mathrm{n} = 1$, it can be readily demonstrated from the above equilibria that

$$K_3 \cdot K_4 = K_1 \cdot K_2 \quad [40]$$

Given the above hypothesis that $K_2 > K_3$ (i.e., the affinity of the receptor for the effector is greater in the presence of hormone), it is evident that $K_4 > K_1$. Thus binding of a hormone by a homogeneous population of receptor molecules can, as suggested by the mobile receptor model, lead to complicated binding kinetics; the complicated binding kinetics predicted by the mobile receptor model (e.g., nonlinear Scatchard plots) might otherwise (incorrectly) be interpreted in terms of a heterogeneity of receptor molecules. In a sense, Eqs. [36] and [39] depict the T and R states, respectively, of the two-state model discussed above.

The mobile receptor model introduces enormous flexibility into the possible actions of hormones and permits a complexity of kinetics (e.g., depending on the values of m and n) that potentially may account for many observed phenomena in connection with hormone effects. It would, as suggested above and depicted in Fig. 8, rationalize the differential modulation of independent membrane processes by a single hormone–receptor complex if the complex exhibited different affinities toward two or more membrane-localized effectors. Furthermore, as developed by De Haën (22), the differential maximal activation of an effector (e.g., adenyl cyclase) common to several hormones could be explained in terms of distinct affinities of the various hormone receptors for the common enzymatic unit. Additionally, the complex α- and β-adrenergic effects of biological systems may be explained in terms of the interactions of multiple receptors with multiple effectors.

An important aspect of the mobile receptor model, not dealt with by the two-state models outlined above, concerns both the levels of effectors and receptors present in a given cell and the receptor/effector ratio that may well vary under different physiological conditions. For example, denervation supersensitivity might be rationalized in terms of variations in the receptor to effector ratio. Alternatively, the ratio of adenyl cyclase effector molecules relative to the total number of receptors for distinct hormone activators would determine whether or not "additivity" of enzymatic activation might be observed for separate hormones.

The detailed mathematical analyses of the mobile receptor model by Jacobs and Cuatrecasas (33) and by De Haën (22) indicate that the binding of a homogeneous ligand with a unique receptor molecule can exhibit nonlinear Scatchard plots, Hill plots consistent with "negative" cooperativity, *and* increased ligand off-rates determined with radiolabeled derivatives in the presence of high concentrations of hormone. By supposing a situation in which there is an excess of receptors (e.g., 10- to 20-fold) compared with effectors, the model can also predict the effect on the ligand-binding data of "spare," but *equivalent* receptors. In such a case, at least two "affinity" sites for the ligand would be detected by binding studies, only one of which "sites" would appear to coincide with the ED_{50} for the biological dose–response curve. All of the receptors would, nonetheless, be equivalent and would contribute to the overall responsiveness of the system.

The above discussion should serve to indicate that the mobile receptor model is sufficiently versatile to account for many, if not all of the observed phenomena concerning hormone action. Moreover, the model is of more than heurisitic value in that the putative existence of effector molecules for certain receptors can be potentially studied in detail. It is to these ends that the more recent studies of ligand binding are directed.

IV. CONCLUSIONS

From the outlines of the various receptor models described in this chapter it is possible to appreciate the enormous but still limited strides that have been made in understanding the detailed mechanisms whereby certain hormones cause a biological response. As experimental expertise has developed (particularly for work over the past decade), the theories have become more explicit in terms of the reacting species. As is the case for the development of any area, several theories have pointed the way to new experimental observations, and in turn, new data, resulting from the development of new techniques, have led to more detailed and explicit models of drug action. As a rule, the newer models provide for the incorporation of most of the aspects of the older ones. On the whole, the various explicit models have focused on the action of agents at the individual cellular level, whereas "response" is generated by the tissue as a whole. However, even if the overall organ response is a summed expression of the sensitivities of responding units in the tissue, as suggested by Gaddum (24) and as developed by Rodbard (42,43), it is expected that the fundamental governing mechanisms will reside at the cellular level, for example, as detailed in the mobile receptor model. It should be emphasized that the receptor mechanisms dealt with in this chapter are clearly biased in terms of the action of neurotransmitters which, like many hormones, initiate their actions via cell surface interactions. The receptor mechanisms involved in the action of agents such as steroid hormones, while perhaps having certain aspects in common with the mechanism of neurotransmitter action, are expected to have other unique features. It will be evident from other chapters in this volume that the challenge of detecting the many specific membrane-localized "recognition" molecules has been largely met, such that one is now faced with the much more onerous task of unraveling the remainder of the receptor mechanisms leading to a cellular response. Hopefully, the various theories, as outlined in this chapter, may serve as a stimulus to further fruitful experiments.

V. SUMMARY

The action of those neurotransmitters and hormones that initiate a biological response via an interaction with the plasma membrane has been discussed in terms of several receptor models. Even relatively elementary considerations of the possible relationships between ligand binding and biological response reveal that the shape of the dose–response curves and the associated ED_{50}'s cannot, without many assumptions (e.g., simple occupancy models), be used to deduce the affinity of the initial ligand–receptor interaction. These considerations underscore the value of direct ligand-binding studies in the elucidation of the mechanisms of neurotransmitter action. A variety of receptor models, in addition to the simple occupancy model, have been dealt with. Such models have arisen from attempts to account for a number of observed pharmacological phenomena, such as the stimulatory action of antagonists or the diminishing action of the repeated application of a single drug. While certain models can account for some of the observed data (e.g., the rate theory accounts for drug antagonism in terms of receptor off-rates, whereas "partial agonists" are rationalized in receptor occupancy models in terms of "efficacy" or "intrinsic activity" factors), no single model appears wholly satisfactory. For neurotransmitters, two-state models, wherein the ionophore is envisioned as being closely linked to the receptor, can account for the observed ionic conductance changes. Nonetheless the mobile or floating receptor model where the receptors are allowed to associate with more than one effector (e.g., ionophore or adenylate cyclase) in the plane of the plasma membrane provides perhaps one of the most general and flexible models for neurotransmitter and hormone action. Taken together, the various receptor models provide a most useful context for the planning and evaluation of the kind of ligand-binding experiments described in this volume.

REFERENCES

1. Ariens, E. J. (1954): Affinity and intrinsic activity in the theory of competitive inhibition. *Arch. Int. Pharmacodyn.*, 99:32–49.
2. Ariens, E. J., and Simonis, A. M. (1964): A molecular basis for drug action. *J. Pharm. Pharmacol.*, 16:137–157, 289–312.
3. Arunlakshana, O., and Schild, H. O. (1959): Some quantitative uses of drug antagonists. *Br. J. Pharmacol.*, 14:48–58.
4. Belleau, B. (1965): Conformational perturbation in relation to the regulation of enzyme and receptor behavior. *Adv. Drug Res.*, 2:89–126.
5. Bennett, V., O'Keefe, E., and Cuatrecasas, P. (1975): Mechanism of action of cholera toxin and the mobile receptor theory of hormone receptor adenylate cyclase interactions. *Proc. Natl. Acad. Sci. USA*, 72:33–37.
6. Birdsall, N. J. M., and Hulme, E. C. (1976): Biochemical studies on muscarinic acetylcholine receptors. *J. Neurochem.*, 27:7–16.
7. Blecher, M. (1976): *Methods in Receptor Research; Methods in Molecular Biology*, Vol. 9, edited by A. I. Laskin and J. A. Last, Parts I and II. Marcel Dekker, New York.
8. Burgen, A. S. V. (1966): The drug receptor complex. *J. Pharm. Pharmacol.*, 18:137–149.
9. Carpenter, G., Lembach, K. J., Morrison, M. M., and Cohen, S. (1975): Characterization of the binding of ^{125}I-labeled epidermal growth factor to human fibroblasts. *J. Biol. Chem.*, 250:4297–4304.
10. Chang, K-J., Jacobs, S., and Cuatrecasas, P. (1975): Quantitative aspects of hormone-receptor interactions of high affinity: Effect of receptor concentration and measurement of dissociation constants of labeled and unlabeled hormones. *Biochim. Biophys. Acta*, 406:294–303.
11. Changeux, J-P., and Podleski, T. (1968): On the excitatory and cooperativity of the electroplax membrane. *Proc. Natl. Acad. Sci. USA*, 59:944–950.

12. Changeux, J-P., Blumenthal, R., Kasai, M., and Podleski, T. (1970): Conformational transitions in the course of membrane excitation. In: *Molecular Properties of Drug Receptors*, edited by R. Porter and M. O'Connor, pp. 197–214. Churchill, London.
13. Clark, A. J. (1926): The reaction between acetylcholine and muscle cells. *J. Physiol. (Lond)*, 61:530–546.
14. Clark, A. J. (1926): The antagonism of acetylcholine by atropine. *J. Physiol. (Lond)*, 61:547–556.
15. Clark, A. J. (1927): The reaction between acetylcholine and muscle cells. Part II. *J. Physiol. (Lond)*, 64:123–143.
16. Clark, A. J. (1937): General Pharmacology. In: *Handbook of Experimental Pharmacology*, Vol. 4. Springer Verlag, Berlin.
17. Colquhoun, D. (1973): The relation between classical and cooperative models for drug action. In: *Drug Receptors*, edited by H.D. Rang, pp. 149–182. University Press, Baltimore.
18. Cuatrecasas, P. (1971): Insulin-receptor interactions in adipose tissue cells: Direct measurement and properties. *Proc. Natl. Acad. Sci. USA*, 68:1264–1268.
19. Cuatrecasas, P. (1974): Membrane receptors. *Annu. Rev. Biochem.*, 43:169–214.
20. Cuatrecasas, P. (1975): Hormone receptors—their function in cell membranes and some problems related to methodology. *Adv. Cyclic Nucleotide Res.*, 5:79–104.
21. Cuatrecasas, P., and Hollenberg, M. D. (1976): Membrane receptors and hormone action. *Adv. Protein Chem.*, 30:251–451.
22. De Haën, C. (1976): The non-stoichiometric floating receptor model for hormone-sensitive adenylate cyclase. *J. Theor. Biol.*, 58:383–400.
23. Devreotes, P. N., Gardner, J. M., and Fambrough, D. M. (1977): Kinetics of biosynthesis of acetylcholine receptor and subsequent incorporation into plasma membrane of cultured chick skeletal muscles. *Cell*, 10:365–373.
24. Gaddum, J. H. (1926): The action of adrenalin and ergotamine on the uterus of the rabbit. *J. Physiol. (Lond)*, 61:141–150.
25. Gaddum, J. H. (1937): The quantitative effects of antagonistic drugs. *J. Physiol. (Lond)*, 89:7P–9P.
26. Gill, E. W. (1965): Drug receptor interactions. *Prog. Med. Chem.*, 4:39–85.
27. Goldstein, A., Aronow, L., and Kalman, S. M. (1974): *Principles of Drug Action*. Wiley, New York.
28. Gordon, A. S., Davis, C. G., Milfay, D., and Diamond, I. (1977): Phosphorylation of acetylcholine receptors by endogenous protein kinase in receptor-enriched membranes of Torpedo california. *Nature (Lond)*, 267:539–540.
29. Hall, Z. W. (1972): Release of neurotransmitters and their interaction with receptors. *Annu. Rev. Biochem.*, 41:925–952.
30. Hollenberg, M. D., and Cuatrecasas, P. (1975): Insulin and epidermal growth factor: Human fibroblast receptors related to DNA synthesis and amino acid transport. *J. Biol. Chem.*, 250:3845–3853.
31. Hollenberg, M. D., and Cuatrecasas, P. (1978): Distinction of receptor from non-receptor interaction in binding studies: Historical and practical perspectives. In: *The Receptors, A Comprehensive Treatise*, edited by R. D. O'Brien, Plenum Press, New York *(in press)*.
32. Hollenberg, M. D., and Gregory, H. (1976): Human urogastrone and mouse epidermal growth factor share a common receptor site in cultured human fibroblasts. *Life Sci.*, 20:267–274.
33. Jacobs, S., and Cuatrecasas, P. (1976): The mobile receptor hypothesis and "cooperativity" of hormone binding application to insulin. *Biochim. Biophys. Acta*, 433:482–495.
34. Kahn, C. R. (1976): Membrane receptors for hormones and neurotransmitters. *J. Cell Biol.*, 70:261–286.
35. Karlin, A. (1967): On the application of a plausible model of allosteric proteins to the receptor for acetylcholine. *J. Theor. Biol.*, 16:306–320.
36. Lefkowitz, R. J. (1975): Identification of adenylate cyclase-coupled beta adrenergic receptors with radiolabeled beta-adrenergic antagonists. *Biochem. Pharmacol.*, 24:1651–1658.
37. Levitzki, A. (1974): Negative cooperativity in clustered receptors as a possible basis for membrane action. *J. Theor. Biol.*, 44:367–372.
38. Monod, J., Wyman, J., and Changeux, J. P. (1965): On the nature of allosteric transitions: A plausible model. *J. Mol. Biol.*, 12:88–118.
39. Paton, W. D. M. (1961): A theory of drug action based on the rate of drug-receptor combination. *Proc. R. Soc. B.* 154:21–69.

40. Paton, W. D. M., and Rang, H. P. (1965): The uptake of atropine and related drugs by intestinal smooth muscle of the guinea pig in relation to acetylcholine receptors. *Proc. R. Soc. B,* 163:1–44.
41. Paton, W. D. M., and Waud, D. R. (1964): A quantitative investigation of the relationship between rate of access of a drug to a receptor and the ratio of onset or offset of action. *Arch. Exp. Pathol. Pharmacol.,* 248:124–143.
42. Rodbard, D. (1973): Mathematics of hormone-receptor interaction. I. Basic principles. In: *Receptors for Reproductive Hormones,* edited by B. W. O'Malley and A. R. Means, pp. 289–342. Plenum Press, New York.
43. Rodbard, D. (1973): Theory of hormone-receptor interactions. III. The endocrine target cell as a quantal response unit, a general control mechanism. In: *Receptors for Reproductive Hormones,* edited by B. W. O'Malley and A. R. Means, pp. 342–364. Plenum Press, New York.
44. Roth, J. (1973): Peptide hormone binding to receptors: A review of direct studies in vitro. *Metabolism,* 22:1059–1073.
45. Schild, H. O. (1949): pAx and competitive drug antagonism. *Br. J. Pharmacol.,* 4:277–280.
46. Stephenson, R. P. (1956): A modification of receptor theory. *Br. J. Pharmacol.,* 11:379–393.
47. Stephenson, R. P., and Barlow, R. B. (1970): Concepts of drug action, quantitative pharmacology and biological assay. In: *A Companion to Medical Studies,* Vol. 2, edited by R. Passmore and J. S. Robson, pp. 3.1–3.19. Blackwell, London.
48. Straus, O. H., and Goldstein, A. J. (1943): Zone behavior of enzymes. *J. Gen. Physiol.,* 26:559–585.
49. Teichberg, V. I., Sobel, A., and Changeux, J-P. (1977): In vitro phosphorylation of the acetylcholine receptor. *Nature (Lond),* 267:540–542.
50. Thron, C. D., and Waud, D. R. (1968): The rate of action of atropine. *J. Pharmacol. Exp. Ther.,* 160:91–105.
51. Waud, D. R. (1968): Pharmacological receptors. *Pharmacol. Rev.,* 20:49–88.

Neurotransmitter Receptor Binding, edited by
H. I. Yamamura et al.
Raven Press, New York © 1978.

3

Criteria for Receptor Identification

David R. Burt

Department of Pharmacology and Experimental Therapeutics, University of Maryland School of Medicine, Baltimore, Maryland 21201

I. INTRODUCTION

The initial or recognition stage of neurotransmitter or drug interaction with biological receptors can be studied in the test tube by binding of suitable radioactive ligands (13,20,33,34). However, in undertaking a binding study, especially one involving a new tissue or a new radioactive ligand, one can all too easily be led astray by insufficient attention to the question of whether or not a particular binding site really represents a physiological or a pharmacological receptor. Every attempt should be made to answer this question before proceeding.

The hypothesis that a given binding site represents the receptor for a drug or a neurotransmitter can be supported by a set of necessary but not sufficient criteria that form the principal topic of this chapter. The important thing to remember in attempting receptor identification is that failure to meet only one criterion, even when all others are met, can cast severe doubt on the identification. Likewise, even when all criteria appear to be met by available data, the possibility remains that additional data (e.g., involving a new drug or new class of drugs) will later disprove the identification. The three basic criteria of saturability and kinetics, distribution, and pharmacology will be discussed first, followed by other issues important in binding studies. Illustrations are rather arbitrarily chosen from studies with which the author is familiar.

II. BASIC CRITERIA

A. Saturability and Kinetics of Binding

In performing binding studies, one soon learns that "everything binds to everything," at least to some extent. Thus it can almost be guaranteed that if tissue is exposed to a radioactive drug, then some binding of radioactivity will occur. A minimal requirement for this binding to be worthy of further study is that there be only a finite number of binding sites of rather high affinity. Exactly what constitutes "high affinity" will depend on context, but for reversible ligands used to study neurotransmitter receptors the term usually refers to dissociation constants in the nanomolar range or lower. Thus in this case, if higher and higher concentrations of radioactive drug are added, then the binding will increase to the point where all sites are occupied but no further; that is, it will saturate.

A more useful way of demonstrating the same phenomenon, especially in initial experiments, is to add to a set of tubes the "blanks," a large excess of the same drug in nonradioactive form. If this addition lowers the amount of radioactivity bound, then, by definition, saturable binding exists. This arises because the addition of nonradioactive drug lowers the specific radioactivity of the drug in the incubation mixture as it raises the total drug concentration. If binding continues to increase in proportion to concentration, which would occur if there are only a large number of very low affinity binding sites, then the bound radioactivity will remain the same. However, if at least one class of binding sites, termed saturable or "specific" sites, becomes fully occupied (saturates), then the reduced drug-specific activity in conjunction with a stable amount of total drug bound will result in a decrease in bound radioactivity.

1. Competition

Another way of describing the same situation is to say that in the presence of a finite number of binding sites, addition of enough nonradioactive drug molecules of the same or of a different drug will result in their competing with radioactive drug molecules for occupation of the limited number of sites. This competition, sometimes referred to as displacement, will reduce the number of bound radioactive drug molecules. The "pharmacology" of the binding, to be discussed in a later section, refers to the relative effectiveness of different drugs in acting as competing agents.

2. Number of Sites

An important question relating to saturability concerns the actual number of binding sites in the tissue under study. Too large a number, usually accompanied by a low affinity, suggests that the binding is not to a receptor. Thus far the maximal densities of neurotransmitter receptor-binding sites in brain regions have tended to fall in the vicinity of 10 to 100 pmoles ligand bound per gram of tissue (34). Values in many peripheral tissues appear to be similar (10,32,39).

The number of sites is also an issue when two or more radioactive ligands are supposed to bind to the same receptor. If all ligands do not yield similar numbers of binding sites, then it is clear that they all cannot be identified with the same receptor, at least without further explanation.

3. Errors

Two errors relating to saturability are sometimes made in studies claiming to have identified a neurotransmitter receptor. The first error is the use of a 100-fold or other arbitrary excess of nonradioactive drug to demonstrate saturability of binding without reference to the dissociation constant. The extent of the excess relative to the concentration of radioactive drug is relevant only when the concentration of radioactive drug is much higher than its dissociation constant of binding. Otherwise the important thing is the extent of the excess relative to the dissociation constant itself. Thus it is customary to use as a blank a concentration of nonradioactive drug equivalent to roughly 100 times or more of the dissociation constant regardless of whether the concentration of radioactive drug is equal to the dissociation constant or whether it is only 1% of the dissociation constant.

The second and more serious error is the claim to have demonstrated "specificity" of binding when all that has been demonstrated is saturability. Saturability is only a minimal criterion for interest, and is many steps removed from a demonstration of specificity, or identification with a given receptor. (The term "specific binding" may still be loosely used as a synonym for saturable binding if the blanks contain a large excess of the same nonradioactive drug as the radioactive one and if it has been demonstrated separately that all of this saturable binding is indeed "specific.") Examples abound in the literature of saturable, relatively high-affinity binding of radioactive drugs to inert materials and to apparently irrelevant tissue sites. Thus insulin binds to talc (12) and radioactive opiates bind to glass fiber filters (36) with affinities in the nanomolar range. Interestingly, in both cases the binding also exhibits a considerable degree of pharmacological specificity, although not exactly matching biological effects. Similarly, radioactive thyrotropin-releasing hormone (TRH) binds to two dissimilar classes of sites in liver and brain with affinities in the low micromolar range (5). Both are distinct from the much higher affinity and less plentiful sites in anterior pituitary and brain that appear to represent TRH receptors, but again the lower affinity sites exhibit a considerable degree of pharmacological specificity for TRH analogs.

4. *Kinetics*

Saturability as discussed thus far has referred to equilibrium measurements of reversible binding reactions. A related criterion for meaningfulness of binding is that it be well behaved kinetically. The equations describing simple binding reactions predict that the equilibrium dissociation constant, whether measured by adding increasing concentrations of radioactive drug (saturation curve) or nonradioactive drug (competition or displacement curve), should also be obtainable as the ratio of the rate constant for dissociation, k_{-1}, over the rate constant for association, k_1.

Failure of this ratio to yield the equilibrium dissociation constant suggests that a complicating factor or artifact has entered the system, for example, that a catecholamine ligand has to undergo oxidation before binding (26,38), that a peptide ligand has to undergo partial degradation before binding, or that there is an unrecognized additional binding site. Ligand modification before binding can also be recognized by checking the identity of bound radioactivity chromatographically and would have the consequence of slowing down the apparent association reaction. Any of these factors would make it extremely doubtful that the binding observed is to the desired receptor.

5. Time Course

The time course of the binding itself may have important implications for specificity when anything is known about the time course of production of biological effect. Since additional steps are involved in a drug's producing a biological effect, the presumption here is that a drug's binding to its receptors, when both are present in appropriate concentrations, should be at least as fast as the appearance of biological effect. This consideration led Paton and Rang (30) to question the receptor identification of the atropine binding sites they observed in smooth muscle in their pioneering study, since the binding of [^{3}H]atropine appeared to be too slow relative to atropine's blockade of acetylcholine-induced contractions.

Similarly, the dissociation of receptor binding should be at least as fast as the "washout" of biological effect. Binding of antagonists thus should not appear irreversible when their biological blockade of neurotransmitter effects is readily reversible. For neurotransmitters themselves, whose actions are in general rapid (time course of seconds to milliseconds), association and dissociation of binding would be expected to be similarly rapid. Higher affinities in general correspond to slower dissociation rates, so that problems may arise in interpreting observed high-affinity binding of neurotransmitters. Thus high-affinity binding of dopamine to calf striatal membranes has a half-life of over a minute (7), whereas dopamine's synaptic actions appear to be terminated in a matter of milliseconds (22). One way around this difficulty is to postulate that the high-affinity binding dopamine site, which has the right pharmacology and distribution, corresponds to a desensitized state of the receptor.

6. Irreversible Ligands

Many of these considerations naturally do not apply to irreversible or essentially irreversible ligands such as alkalating agents or α-bungarotoxin and related toxins used to study the junctional nicotinic acetylcholine receptor (23,29,32). Here, the effect of competing drugs on the rate of association of toxin binding is the best measure of pharmacological specificity, since in theory true equilibrium is not reached until all binding sites are occupied by toxin or until all toxin molecules are bound (9).

B. Distribution of Binding Sites

Once a high-affinity, saturable binding site has been detected, presumably with some preliminary pharmacological data to relate it to a given neurotransmitter receptor, the next question to ask is whether binding of the same characteristics is present only where receptors for the neurotransmitter are known to exist. This question commonly involves three kinds of distribution study: among tissues, among brain regions, and among subcellular fractions.

1. *Tissue Distribution*

The experiment here is simply to survey many different organs or tissues, looking for binding resembling that already tentatively identified with a neurotransmitter receptor. Such binding may not be detectable in all tissues known to be innervated with the transmitter, but at least it should not be found where the transmitter is known to be absent.

2. *Brain Regional Distribution and Correlation with Presynaptic Markers*

The experiment is again a survey; the interpretation can be extended to attempt to relate the density of binding sites in a brain region to the density of innervation of that region by neurons using the relevant neurotransmitter. The "density of innervation" must be derived from independent studies of levels of the neurotransmitter and of its synthetic enzymes, of metabolites, of high-affinity uptake sites and other presynaptic markers. It should be noted that because of problems of differential localization of these presynaptic markers to cell bodies versus nerve terminals and of the existence of different sizes and types of nerve terminals using the same transmitter, it cannot be expected that all markers will correlate exactly with each other, let alone with postsynaptic neurotransmitter receptors. Moreover, there is no reason why the number of neurons receiving nerve terminals using a given transmitter in a brain region has to be proportional to the actual number of those terminals in the region. The number of receptors in a region may depend more on the number of neurons possessing them than on the number of synapses those neurons receive. Synapses themselves may vary in size and in the number of receptors associated with each. Finally, the receptor type under study may be only one of several responding to a given neurotransmitter (e.g., α and β for norepinephrine, muscarinic and nicotinic for acetylcholine). In spite of all these qualifications, a rough correlation between density of binding sites and various presynaptic markers can be expected in most tissues or brain regions.

3. *Subcellular Distribution*

The distribution of binding among subcellular fractions of brain is perhaps the least informative of the types of distribution study unless the subcellular fractionation scheme is very refined. Brain fractions are always impure, cross-contaminated and derived from a variety of cell types. Thus the binding will always tend to be rather widely distributed among fractions. Moreover, it can always be argued that inappropriately localized binding sites are in the process of synthesis or degradation. Nonetheless, binding should be highest in fractions demonstrated to contain "synaptic membranes," although the degree to which these are postsynaptic, as opposed to presynaptic, is usually not clear. The localization of binding to synaptic membranes does not exclude the possibility that a membrane-bound enzyme, uptake site, storage site, or other nonreceptor macromolecule is the binding site and does not specifically associate the binding site with any given neurotransmitter.

4. *Presence of Response*

Regardless of whether or not direct neuroanatomical or biochemical evidence suggests the presence of appropriate innervation in a tissue or brain region possessing binding sites, it would seem essential to have at least some pharmacological evidence for receptors, that is, that the tissue is somehow responsive to the neurotransmitter or related agents or that the brain region possesses some neurons that respond electrically to application of the neurotransmitter or related agents. Correlating the presence of a response with the presence of binding is most clear-cut in a system consisting of only one cell type such as a clonal cell line. Thus β-adrenergic receptor binding has been found only in cell lines with β-stimulated adenylate cyclase activity (27).

5. *Binding without Function*

What does it mean if binding with appropriate saturability and pharmacology is observed in a tissue where there is no evidence of innervation or of pharmacological response? Such otherwise promising binding sites in search of a function have been termed "acceptors" (4,30). Several interpretations are possible. The most optimistic is that previous experiments have somehow missed the innervation or the response of the tissue to the neurotransmitter, either by not looking at all or by looking for the wrong response. Another possibility, especially attractive for binding to liver membranes, is that the binding is to a degradative enzyme whose specificity happens to resemble that of a receptor. Related possibilities include binding to storage and uptake sites. Finally, the binding may be to true receptor molecules that have become uncoupled from any response and thus represent developmental or evolutionary "leftovers." An example is the persistence of β-adrenergic receptor binding on rat reticulocytes as they mature into red blood cells (3). This occurs during the same period when the reticulocytes are rapidly losing their β-stimulated adenylate cyclase activity.

C. Pharmacology of Binding

A receptor is defined or identified in the first place in terms of its pharmacology. Thus the most important criterion in identifying a binding site with a neurotransmitter receptor is the detailed pharmacology of the binding. On a relative basis, this means that drugs that are effective in mimicking or blocking the effects of the neurotransmitter should compete for binding at low concentrations, whereas ineffective drugs should compete only at very high concentrations if at all. Ideally, the pharmacology of the binding should correlate quantitatively with the pharmacology of receptor-mediated effects for a large number of drugs of different types.

It is important to emphasize at this point that "specificity," in the sense that drugs of different structures do not compete for binding, is not a sufficient pharmacological criterion of receptor identification. This type of behavior may be expected for any relatively high-affinity binding site. The correlation with biological effects is the important consideration.

1. Quantitative Correlation

In practice, quantitative correlation with receptor-mediated effects is difficult to achieve. Often the major problems arise not from the binding experiments themselves, but rather from the nature of the other pharmacological data with which the binding data are being compared. Clearly, in measuring the *in vivo* response to a drug, particularly a behavioral response, the experimenter is dealing with many more variables than just the affinity of the drug for its receptor.

Variables are reduced by applying drugs by microiontophoresis and measuring responses of individual neurons. This situation, although yielding good comparative data among drugs, is very difficult to quantify. Successful correlation of binding and pharmacological data is most likely to be achieved where the pharmacological response, like the binding, is measured *in vitro,* preferably under conditions identical to the binding. Prominent examples of *in vitro* measurements include the effects of neurotransmitters on smooth muscle contraction and on adenylate cyclase activity. Excellent correlations have been reported between measurements of stimulation and blockade of β-receptor-stimulated adenylate cyclase activity and measurements of competition for [^{3}H]dihydroalprenolol binding, for example (28). Similar success has been achieved in correlating opiate receptor binding affinities with effectiveness in inhibiting or blocking inhibition of electrically induced contractions of guinea pig ileum (10) and in correlating muscarinic receptor-binding affinities with effectiveness in inhibiting acetylcholine-induced contractions of guinea pig ileum (2,35,39). As will be discussed further in Chapter 8, receptor binding has even proved capable in some cases of predicting *in vivo* behavioral responses to drugs such as antischizophrenics (11).

2. Agonists and Antagonists

Apparent binding affinities typically differ according to whether an agonist (such as the neurotransmitter itself) or an antagonist has been used as radioactive ligand, complicating attempts to correlate binding affinities with biological potencies. These findings have been explained variously in terms of preferential binding of agonists and antagonists to different receptor conformational states (33), including preferential binding of agonists to desensitized receptors, and in terms of multiple classes of agonist binding sites (2). Moreover, because of steps intervening between receptor occupation and production of biological effects, there are difficulties in interpreting biological potencies of agonists that do not exist for antagonists (13). The result is that only the affinities of antagonists competing for antagonist binding regularly match their biological potencies.

For purposes of the present discussion, it is sufficient to note these differences and to realize that it is usually necessary to settle for comparing relative affinities of agonists with biological potencies. Thus muscarinic agonists are two to three orders of magnitude less potent in competing for antagonist [^{3}H]quinuclidinyl benzilate binding in membrane preparations of guinea pig ileum longitudinal muscle than in contracting the intact muscle (35,39) whereas dopaminergic agonists are approximately two orders of magnitude more potent in competing for agonist [^{3}H]dopamine binding in membrane preparations of calf striatum than in stimulating adenylate cyclase activity in homogenates of rat striatum (8). However, in both cases the relative binding affinities appear to be in agreement with the relative biological potencies.

3. Stereospecificity

One of the most useful types of pharmacological criterion in identifying receptor binding is stereospecificity. Stereospecificity may involve either the radioactive ligand itself or nonradioactive drugs used as competing agents. Many responses of biological systems distinguish between stereoisomers of drugs. Clearly, binding to neurotransmitter receptors mediating these responses should do the same. Thus one of the major and too long ignored items of evidence that direct catecholamine binding (as studied until very recently) could not represent β-adrenergic receptors was its lack of stereospecificity (24,37).

Although stereospecificity of binding is extremely useful, it does not constitute absolute proof of receptor identification. The clearest illustration is the demonstration of stereospecific binding of opiates to glass fiber filters (36) and cerebrosides (25). Likewise, the dopamine receptor appears capable of limited discrimination between the stereoisomers of epinephrine and norepinephrine, usually taken to be characteristic of adrenergic receptors, and of excellent discrimination between the stereoisomers of lysergic acid diethylamide (LSD), initially thought to be characteristic of serotonin receptors (7). Conversely, the serotonin receptor appears capable of distinguishing stereoisomers of butaclamol, an important property of dopamine receptors (1,16). No doubt nonreceptor proteins (e.g., metabolic enzymes) in some instances are similarly capable of differentially binding stereoisomers of drugs used to label receptors.

4. Multiple Sites

The pharmacology of binding becomes particularly important when attempts are made to use a radioactive ligand that binds to multiple classes of sites, only one of which represents the receptor of interest. This situation is typical.

Moreover, many centrally acting drugs, such as LSD (6), will bind to more than one receptor type as well as to nonreceptor sites. The receptors must then be identified and be distinguished on pharmacological grounds using drugs that are more (or differently) specific than the radioactive ligand itself.

5. *Choice of Blank*

With multiple sites, a critical factor in identifying the receptor of interest is making the right choice of blank. Using a very large excess of the same drug in nonradioactive form is inappropriate since this will compete for all classes of binding sites. Rather a carefully chosen excess of the neurotransmitter itself is often the best choice, although other highly specific drugs (e.g., stereoisomers) may be attractive alternatives.

6. *Lack of Additivity*

Where two or more drugs are available as blanks, and blanks are relatively high, an important criterion for identifying the portion of total binding representing receptor binding is to show that maximally effective concentrations of both drugs compete for the same portion of total binding whether they are added individually or in combination. Thus stereospecific displacement of [^{3}H]haloperidol binding to calf caudate membranes by (+)—butaclamol and displacement by dopamine both represent approximately 40% of the total binding and are not additive, an important part of the evidence that both drugs are competing for the same class of [^{3}H]haloperidol binding sites that represent dopamine receptors (7). In theory, for a situation involving multiple sites, lack of additivity with the blank should be shown for each drug that is investigated.

7. *Noncompetitive Agents*

Chemical or enzymatic modification of receptors may be expected to affect biological responses in the same way as it does receptor binding. This becomes another useful pharmacological criterion for receptor identification, especially when biological responsiveness can be measured under the same conditions as binding. Thus part of the evidence that nicotinic acetylcholine receptors can be identified by reversible binding of radioactive acetylcholine as well as by irreversible neurotoxin binding is the observation that the effects of sulfhydryl reagents on acetylcholine binding to particulate preparations of torpedo electroplax, as measured by equilibrium dialysis, resemble the effects of these agents on acetylcholine-induced depolarization of innervated membranes of eel electroplax (14).

8. *Antibodies*

Specific antibodies may provide another pharmacological tool in receptor identification when a receptor has been purified from one tissue and its identity is being established in another. Thus nicotinic receptors at the mammalian neuromuscular junction have been shown to resemble closely those in fish electric organs by the production of a myasthenia gravis-like autoimmune syndrome in rabbits by antibodies to purified acetylcholine receptors from electric organs (31).

9. Response to Radioactive Ligands

Another aspect of the pharmacology of binding as a criterion for receptor identification has to do with the presence of a pharmacological response of the tissue under study to the radioactive ligand used in the binding experiments. That such a response should exist is important for three reasons. The first reason is purely methodological and is particularly relevant when the ligand has been modified (e.g., by iodination) in order to make it radioactive. Then it is necessary to demonstrate that the modified ligand has retained biological activity. The second reason has already been mentioned in the section on distribution of binding and deals in part with the question of whether or not receptors should be expected where binding has been found. The third reason is related to the second and addresses the question of whether the proper ligand is being used to label a given receptor when it is known that the receptor is present and that the same ligand has labeled similar receptors in other tissues.

This situation arises in the use of α-bungarotoxin to attempt to label nicotinic acetylcholine receptors in sympathetic ganglia. Ganglia are known to contain nicotinic receptors that are pharmacologically distinct from those at the neuromuscular junction (18). Junctional receptors have been labeled with great success by α-bungarotoxin and related toxins (23,29,32) and binding of somewhat similar characteristics has been described in sympathetic ganglia (17,19). The problem is that electrophysiological studies have failed to demonstrate any blockade by α-bungarotoxin of nicotinic responses of ganglion cells to acetylcholine (21). Ganglia thus seem to contain α-bungarotoxin binding sites, for which cholinergic agents compete, that are distinct from at least some of their nicotinic receptors.

III. OTHER IMPORTANT ISSUES

A. Tissue Linearity

Tissue linearity is important in binding studies to demonstrate the absence of artifacts, such as receptor or ligand degradation during the incubation and unrecognized endogenous ligands. Although a minor degree of downward curvature in graphs plotting binding against added tissue is unlikely to lead to an incorrect receptor identification, it will certainly yield incorrect or ambiguous values for such parameters as densities of binding sites. Thus it is always desirable to find conditions that will give linearity of binding with tissue even if this entails one or more membrane purification steps and a lowering of recovery of receptors. The rarer condition of upward curvature in tissue linearity graphs, which is equally undesirable, may indicate an inappropriate choice of blank or loss of some binding sites during their separation from free ligand.

B. Temperature Dependence

Temperature in the range of 0 to 37° C will strongly affect the rates of association and dissociation of binding reactions and may affect equilibrium dissociation constants. Although this type of data is capable of yielding useful information about energy barriers and receptor mechanisms, it is rarely critical in receptor identification.

An exception is that preincubation of tissue or running incubations themselves at temperatures much above 40° C should decrease and ultimately destroy receptor binding. At higher temperatures the complex tertiary structure of receptor proteins becomes more and more disrupted until finally the receptor is heat denatured. Maintained or increased binding at high temperatures suggests the possibility of a covalent chemical reaction of the radioactive ligand or a breakdown product rather than reversible receptor binding. This appeared to be the case for nonreceptor "binding" of [^{3}H]epinephrine to proteins from rat heart (38).

A further technical consideration in initial experiments is that a strong dependence of binding on temperature in the normal range suggests that what is being measured is a rate process such as active uptake rather than an equilibrium binding reaction. Efforts to assess this possibility, such as using high ligand concentrations and long incubations, are then indicated.

C. Effects of pH and Ions

Neurotransmitter receptors, as surface membrane proteins, operate normally under conditions of physiological pH. Thus, in the absence of other knowledge, it may be anticipated that the pH maxima of neurotransmitter receptor binding will be near 7.4. Exceptions will presumably reflect response maxima that differ from pH 7.4 or else extraneous factors such as solubility or stability of the ligand. As in the case of high temperatures, extremes of pH should reduce or eliminate binding as the structure of receptors is disrupted.

Effects of ions are less predictable. Certainly receptor binding should at least exist in the presence of physiological concentrations of ions. But whether it will be maximal, let alone detectable, under these conditions depends on other circumstances. One problem arises from the existence of sodium-dependent high-affinity uptake sites for many neurotransmitters in brain, both in nerve terminals themselves and in glia. Thus in order to detect binding of [^{3}H]γ-aminobutyric acid (GABA) to GABA receptors, it is necessary to exclude sodium from the incubation to aid in reducing binding to much more numerous sodium-dependent (presumably uptake) sites (15).

Effects of ions on binding can aid in receptor identification when the effects of receptor activation on ionic conductances are known and there is close or direct coupling between the receptor binding site and the "ionic conductance modulator." Thus part of the evidence that [^{3}H]strychnine binding to spinal cord membranes represents synaptic glycine receptors is that the ability of various anions to substitute for chloride in mediating glycine-induced synaptic inhibition parallels their potency relative to chloride in inhibiting strychnine binding (40).

D. Identity of Bound Radioactivity

An important demonstration in binding studies with a new radioactive ligand is that most or all of the bound radioactivity still represents the original ligand. Usually there will be some other indication that the ligand is undergoing chemical or enzymatic modification during the incubation, such as a slow time course, a decrease in binding at longer times, or a lack of tissue linearity. Nonetheless, verification of the identity of bound radioactivity remains an important part of receptor identification. Where this proves difficult or impossible, verification of the identity of unbound radioactivity after prolonged incubation may provide a minimal substitute.

IV. CONCLUSIONS

Final proof of receptor identification requires purification of the binding site and the demonstration that adding the purified binding site, perhaps with other components, to model membrane systems results in their gaining receptor properties. However, by demonstrating that a binding site satisfies all of the criteria discussed in this chapter, one can make it extremely difficult to come up with any explanation of his findings other than that he has identified a neurotransmitter receptor.

V. SUMMARY

A binding site may be identified as a receptor for a drug or neurotransmitter only after a careful comparison of the properties of the binding site with the properties expected of the receptor. Thus the binding site should be present in limited numbers and have a suitably high affinity (saturability), should bind the radioactive ligand and lose the binding at least as fast as the rates of production and loss of biological effects of the ligand (kinetics), should be found only where receptors are expected and not be found elsewhere (distribution), and should be occupied only by drugs effective at the receptor at concentrations in proportion to those needed to produce a biological effect (pharmacology). In addition, the binding at the site should be destroyed by high temperatures (temperature sensitivity) and other manipulations that affect binding should similarly affect the appearance of biological effects. An exact matching of binding properties with expected receptor properties argues strongly for a receptor identification for the binding site.

ACKNOWLEDGMENTS

The author would like to thank Dr. M. E. Eldefrawi for useful comments on the manuscript. While working on this chapter, the author was supported in part by USPHS grant 1 R01 MH29671.

VI. REFERENCES

1. Bennett, J. P., Jr., and Snyder, S. H. (1976): Serotonin and lysergic acid diethylamide binding in rat brain membranes: Relationship to postsynaptic serotonin receptors. *Mol. Pharmacol.,* 12:373–389.
2. Birdsall, N. J. M., and Hulme, E. C. (1976): Biochemical studies on muscarinic acetylcholine receptors. *J. Neurochem.,* 27:7–16.
3. Bilezikian, J. P., Spiegel, A. M., Brown, E. M., and Aurbach, G. D. (1977): Identification and persistence of beta adrenergic receptors during maturation of the rat reticulocyte. *Mol. Pharmacol.,* 13:775–785.
4. Birnbaumer, L., Pohl, S. L., and Kaumann, A. J. (1974): Receptors and acceptors: A necessary distinction in hormone binding studies. *Adv. Cyclic Nucleotide Res.,* 4:239–281.
5. Burt, D. R., and Snyder, S. H. (1975): Thyrotropin releasing hormone (TRH): Apparent receptor binding in rat brain membranes. *Brain Res.,* 93:309–328.
6. Burt, D. R., Creese, I., and Snyder, S. H. (1976): Binding interactions of lysergic acid diethylamide and related agents with dopamine receptors in the brain. *Mol. Pharmacol.,* 12:631–638.
7. Burt, D. R., Creese, I., and Snyder, S. H. (1976): Properties of [^{3}H]haloperidol and [^{3}H]dopamine binding associated with dopamine receptors in calf brain membranes. *Mol. Pharmacol.,* 12:800–812.
8. Burt, D. R., Enna, S. J., Creese, I., and Snyder, S. H. (1975): Dopamine receptor binding in the corpus striatum of mammalian brain. *Proc. Natl. Acad. Sci. USA,* 72:4655–4659.
9. Colquhoun, D., and Rang, H. P. (1976): Effects of inhibitors on the binding of iodinated α-bungarotoxin to acetylcholine receptors in rat muscle. *Mol. Pharmacol.,* 12:519–535.
10. Creese, I., and Snyder, S. H. (1975): Opiate receptor binding and pharmacological activity in the guinea pig intestine. *J. Pharmacol. Exp. Ther.,* 194:205–219.
11. Creese, I., Burt, D. R., and Snyder, S. H. (1976): Dopamine receptor binding predicts clinical and pharmacological potencies of antischizophrenic drugs. *Science,* 192:481–483.
12. Cuatrecasas, P., and Hollenberg, M. D. (1975): Binding of insulin and other hormones to non-receptor materials: Saturability, specificity and apparent "negative cooperativity." *Biochem. Biophys. Res. Commun.,* 62:31–41.
13. Cuatrecasas, P., and Hollenberg, M. D. (1976): Membrane receptors and hormone action. *Adv. Protein Chem.,* 30:251–451.
14. Eldefrawi, M. E., and Eldefrawi, A. T. (1972): Characterization and partial purification of the acetylcholine receptor from Torpedo electroplax. *Proc. Natl. Acad. Sci. USA,* 69:1776–1780.
15. Enna, S. J., and Snyder, S. H. (1975): Properties of γ-aminobutyric acid (GABA) receptor binding in rat brain synaptic membrane fractions. *Brain Res.,* 100:81–97.
16. Enna, S. J., Bennett, J. P., Jr., Burt, D. R., Creese, I., and Snyder, S. H. (1976): Stereospecificity of interaction of neuroleptic drugs with neurotransmitters and correlation with clinical potency. *Nature (Lond.),* 263:338–341.
17. Fumagalli, L., De Renzis, G., and Miani, N. (1976): Acetylcholine receptors: Number and distribution in intact and deafferented superior cervical ganglion of the rat. *J. Neurochem.,* 27:47–52.
18. Goodman, L. S., and Gilman, A. G., editors (1975): *The Pharmacological Basis of Therapeutics,* 5th ed., Chaps. 27 and 28. Macmillan, New York.
19. Greene, L. A., Sytkowski, A. J., Vogel, Z., and Nirenberg, M. W. (1973): α-Bungarotoxin used as a probe for acetylcholine receptors of cultured neurones. *Nature (Lond.),* 243:163–166.
20. Kahn, C. R. (1976): Membrane receptors for hormones and neurotransmitters. *J. Cell Biol.,* 70:261–286.

21. Ko, C-P., Burton, H., and Bunge, R. P. (1976): Synaptic transmission between rat spinal cord explants and dissociated superior cervical ganglion neurons in tissue culture. *Brain Res.*, 117:437–460.
22. Krnjevic, K. (1975): Electrophysiology of dopamine receptors. In: *Adv. Neurol.*, 9:13–24.
23. Lee, C. Y. (1972): Chemistry and pharmacology of polypeptide venoms in snake toxins. *Annu. Rev. Pharmacol.*, 12:265–286.
24. Lefkowitz, R. J. (1975): Identification of adenylate cyclase-coupled beta-adrenergic receptors with radiolabeled beta-adrenergic antagonists. *Biochem. Pharmacol.*, 24:1651–1658.
25. Loh, H. H., Cho, T. M., Wu, Y. C., and Way, E. L. (1974): Stereospecific binding of narcotics to brain cerebrosides. *Life Sci.*, 14:2231–2245.
26. Maguire, M. E., Goldmann, P. H., and Gilman, A. G. (1974): The reaction of [^{3}H]norepinephrine with particulate fractions of cells responsive to catecholamines. *Mol. Pharmacol.*, 10:563–581.
27. Maguire, M. E., Wiklund, R. A., Anderson, H. J., and Gilman, A. G. (1976): Binding of [^{125}I]iodohydroxybenzylpindolol to putative β-adrenergic receptors of rat glioma cells and other cell clones. *J. Biol. Chem.*, 251:1221–1231.
28. Mukherjee, C., Caron, M. G., Mullikin, D., and Lefkowitz, R. J. (1976): Structure-activity relationships of adenylate cyclase-coupled beta adrenergic receptors: Determination by direct binding studies. *Mol. Pharmacol.*, 12:16–31.
29. O'Brien, R. D., Eldefrawi, M. E., and Eldefrawi, A. T. (1972): Isolation of acetylcholine receptors. *Annu. Rev. Pharmacol.*, 12:19–34.
30. Paton, W. D. M., and Rang, H. P. (1965): The uptake of atropine and related drugs by intestinal smooth muscle of the guinea pig in relation to acetylcholine receptors. *Proc. R. Soc. Lond.* [*Biol.*], 163:1–44.
31. Patrick, J., and Lindstrom, J. (1973): Autoimmune response to acetylcholine receptor. *Science*, 180:871–872.
32. Rang, H. P. (1975): Acetylcholine receptors. *Q. Rev. Biophys.*, 7:283–399.
33. Snyder, S. H. (1975): Neurotransmitter and drug receptors in the brain. *Biochem. Pharmacol.*, 24:1371–1374.
34. Snyder, S. H., and Bennett, J. P., Jr. (1976): Neurotransmitter receptors in the brain: Biochemical identification. *Annu. Rev. Physiol.*, 38:153–175.
35. Snyder, S. H., Chang, K. J., Kuhar, M. J., and Yamamura, H. I. (1975): Biochemical identification of the mammalian muscarinic cholinergic receptor. *Fed. Proc.*, 34:1915–1921.
36. Snyder, S. H., Pasternak, G. W., and Pert, C. B. (1975): Opiate receptor mechanisms. In: *Handbook of Psychopharmacology*, Vol. 5, edited by L. L. Iversen, S. D. Iversen, and S. H. Snyder, pp. 329–360. Plenum Press, New York.
37. Wolfe, B. B., Harden, T. K., and Molinoff, P. B. (1977): In vitro study of β-adrenergic receptors. *Annu. Rev. Pharmacol. Toxicol.*, 17:575–604.
38. Wolfe, B. B., Zirrolli, J. A., and Molinoff, P. B. (1974): Binding of dl-[^{3}H]epinephrine to proteins of rat ventricular muscle: Nonidentity with beta adrenergic receptors. *Mol. Pharmacol.*, 10:582–596.
39. Yamamura, H. I., and Snyder, S. H. (1975): Muscarinic cholinergic receptor binding in the longitudinal muscle of the guinea pig ileum with [^{3}H]quinuclidinyl benzilate. *Mol. Pharmacol.*, 10:861–867.
40. Young, A. B., and Snyder, S. H. (1974): The glycine synaptic receptor: Evidence that strychnine binding is associated with the ionic conductance mechanism. *Proc. Natl. Acad. Sci. USA*, 71:4002–4005.

Neurotransmitter Receptor Binding, edited by
H. I. Yamamura et al.
Raven Press, New York © 1978.

4

Methods in Binding Studies

James P. Bennett Jr.

Department of Pharmacology and Experimental Therapeutics, The Johns Hopkins University School of Medicine, Baltimore, Maryland 21205

I. INTRODUCTION

The purpose of this chapter is to describe in some detail many of the practical aspects of receptor-binding studies. The rapid proliferation of receptor-binding studies gives testimony to the many insights available from what, for the most part, are relatively simple techniques. However, each step in a receptor-binding study is subject to artifact. In part, such artifacts are somewhat unique to receptor-binding studies because of the kinetic restraints imposed by reversible ligand-binding site interactions.

The author will attempt to serve two major purposes in this chapter. First, for those who wish to attempt receptor-binding studies using established ligands and tissues, the methodology (and precautions) presented should be sufficient to allow a successful first experiment. Second, an attempt will be made to couple theoretical aspects of receptor–ligand interactions (cf. Chapters 2 and 3) and the practicalities of experimental detail such that those attempting receptor studies with novel ligands and/or tissues will be guided in their efforts.

The majority of the experimental detail will involve ligands used for mammalian central nervous system neurotransmitter receptors. However, when appropriate for purposes of illustration, receptor research dealing with hormones and receptors outside the CNS, ligands representing possible novel neurotransmitters or neuromodulators within the CNS, and hormones with established peripheral target tissues will also be discussed. Thus the inclusion of a particular ligand in this chapter does not represent an endorsement of that substance as a neurotransmitter substance meeting established neurophysiological and neurochemical criteria (40). However, it is interesting that establishing specific CNS receptor sites for a putative synaptically active substance may now offer ancillary evidence for a true synaptic function. Finally, the nicotinic cholinergic receptor of invertebrate nervous tissue will not be discussed in detail since the literature dealing with this subject is already very extensive (6,7,14,26).

II. THE BINDING EXPERIMENT: PRACTICAL AND THEORETICAL CONSIDERATIONS

A. The Ligand

1. Radioligand

The vast majority of receptor-labeling studies involve binding a radioactive form of either the neurotransmitter/hormone itself or a biologically active analog (agonist), or an appropriate antagonist to membrane preparations (particulate or solubilized) or, in certain cases, to cytoplasmic preparations (i.e., steroid receptors) of target tissues. Thus the first and most critical step in any receptor study is to acquire a radiolabeled ligand of sufficient radiochemical specific activity, purity, stability, and biological activity. Because most receptor sites have equilibrium dissociation constants for ligands in the nanomolar range and below, the particular radioisotope utilized must have a specific activity sufficient to allow accurate measurement of low concentrations. The isotope most commonly used is tritium, which is incorporated into molecules either by direct synthesis or by catalytically induced tritium exchange with hydrogen atoms in the molecular structure. Advantages of tritium labeling include: (a) The labeled product is biologically indistinguishable from the native compound. (b) High specific activities can be obtained (in some cases upward of 30 Ci/mmol). (c) Purification of labeled ligand is simplified since it behaves in a manner identical to the unlabeled compound in analytical systems. (d) With proper storage conditions most tritiated compounds are stable for many months. (e) Tritium has a long radiochemical half-life (greater than 12 years). The disadvantages of tritium labeling include: (a) The fact that very few laboratories possess facilities for tritium labeling and thus the major sources are commercial suppliers, (b) the high initial expense for custom tritiation, and (c) the variable specific activities and radiochemical purities.

For molecules possessing an aromatic hydroxyl group, usually tyrosine residues in a peptide, [^{125}I] can usually be easily incorporated to very high specific activity (upward of 2,000 Ci/mmol) without significant loss of biological activity. For most molecules thus labeled and utilized in receptor-binding studies, monoiodinated compounds usually possess biological activity near or equal to the parent compound whereas diiodinated compounds possess very little if any biological activity. Radioiodination, when appropriate, offers a rapid, convenient, and inexpensive means to generate radiolabeled ligands very suitable for receptor research. The major problems with radioiodinated ligands include: (a) generation of "damaged" but labeled molecules during the iodination procedure, (b) greater susceptibility to radiation-induced destruction of molecular structure (decay catastrophe), (c) different behavior of the iodinated substance in analytical systems compared to the parent molecule, and (d) short radiochemical half-life of ^{125}I (67 days).

Most radioiodinations can be carried out at neutral pH at room temperature using carrier-free sodium ^{125}I and a mild oxidizing agent (chloramine-T, lactoperoxidase plus hydrogen peroxide) (9,12,18,36,37). Typical reaction times are of the order of 30 sec to several minutes with the frequency of diiodination increasing in most instances with longer reaction times. The reactions are stopped by adding a mild reducing agent (i.e., sodium metabisulfite) and free ^{125}I is then separated from iodinated ligand. This separation can be easily accomplished by adsorption of many substances (i.e., peptides) to inert matrices such as talc, microfine quartz crystals, silica, and so forth, and separation by centrifugation. Another very popular method of separation involves gel filtration using molecular sieves (Bio-Gel®, Sephadex®) to separate larger molecules from free ^{125}I. In many cases such simple procedures will yield very pure (greater than 90%) products; but in all cases, the purity of the radioligand and its specific activity must be assayed.

Because most receptor–ligand studies are designed to take place in "zone A" (35), that is, 10% or less of the total ligand available in the incubation solution is bound at equilibrium, radiochemical purity of ligands assumes major importance. The most convenient methods of assaying radioligand purity involve chromatography of one kind or another. Thin layer chromatography (TLC) is usually the most rapid technique and will serve both as an analytical and a preparative procedure. The nature of the solid supports and developing solvent systems used will vary from one substance to another. Several comprehensive reference works are available for TLC procedures (25,34).

Experience indicates that it is best for the individual investigator to determine radiochemical purity himself even on commercially prepared radioligands. Unknown factors such as temperature extremes in shipping (excessive heat or freeze–thaw cycles) and variability in quality control mandate that the investigator analyze radioligands soon after arrival. The need for such analysis after custom tritiation or synthesis is obvious.

In establishing the degree of purity, it is essential to account for total dpm's applied to the assay system (i.e., the TLC plate). A significant percentage of radioactivity in the ligand solution may be present as tritiated solvent that would evaporate during analysis of the chromatogram, yielding a falsely high degree of purity of the total sample. Once radiochemical purity has been established in at least two separate systems, it will be obvious whether or not further purification is necessary. Because of the small percentage of total added radioligand that is bound in most receptor studies, ligands need to be 90% pure at the absolute minimum with a desirable lower limit of 95%. Purification can usually utilize one of the analytical systems "scaled up" to handle a larger sample such as preparative TLC.

After the desired purity is obtained, the radioligand must be assayed to determine specific activity and stored in such a fashion as to minimize decomposition. Most manufacturers will determine the specific activity of each lot of commercially available radioligands as well as the radiochemical purity. Manufacturers' estimates of specific activity are usually accurate and this determination need not be repeated routinely. If there are significant deviations between manufacturers' claims of purity and individual investigators' analyses of purity, then the investigator is obliged to determine specific activity if he decides to purify and use that particular lot of radioligand. Specific activity determinations involve determining the amount of radioactivity present in a given weight or molar unit of compound. The limiting factor in such determinations is usually an analytical method sensitive enough to detect very small quantities of ligand. Examples of methods utilized include uv and/or fluorescence spectrophotometry, gas chromatography, and radioimmunoassay.

Proper radioligand storage is crucial if reproducible results are to be obtained. Light- and oxygen-sensitive compounds must be protected by storage in the dark and in the presence of suitable antioxidants (N_2 atmosphere, ascorbic acid, dithiothreitol). The most common cause of nonoxidative radioligand decomposition in storage is some form of decay catastrophe that is more common with compounds labeled to high specific activity. This deterioration can usually be reduced by (a) including a free radical scavanging solvent such as ethanol or methanol, (b) storing the radioligand as dilutely as feasible, and (c) storing the radioligand solution at as low a temperature as possible without freezing, or storing frozen at −70° C or below in small aliquots such that freeze–thaw cycles will be avoided. Manufacturers will advise on optimum storage conditions.

For radioligands prepared by radioisotope addition (i.e., [^{125}I]-peptides), it is desirable to demonstrate biological activity of the radioiodinated material unless this information has already been demonstrated for the particular ligand. The nature of the bioassay will depend on the hormone labeled and may require large quantities of radioligand compared to the amounts needed in typical binding assays.

B. The Binding Experiment

1. General Considerations

Receptor-binding studies usually follow kinetics very similar to those of classic enzyme–substrate interactions. For reversible ligand–receptor interactions where [R] = concentration of unoccupied receptor sites, [L] = concentration of free ligand, [RL] = concentration of receptor–ligand complex

$$a[R] + b[L] \underset{k_{-1}}{\overset{k_1}{\rightleftharpoons}} c[RL] \qquad [1]$$

describes a general reversible binding phenomenon with a, b, and c representing the stoichiometry of the reaction. At equilibrium, or "steady state," the rate of the forward reaction equals the rate of the reverse reaction

$$k_1[R]^a[L]^b = k_{-1}[RL]^c \qquad [2]$$

The equilibrium binding constant may then be defined either as an association binding constant (K_A)

$$K_A = \frac{k_1}{k_{-1}} = \frac{[RL]^c}{[R]^a[L]^b} \qquad [3]$$

or as a dissociation binding constant (K_D)

$$K_D = \frac{k_{-1}}{k_1} = \frac{[R]^a[L]^b}{[RL]^c} \qquad [4]$$

Thus experimental determination of equilibrium binding affinity constants for reversible reactions requires that experiments be performed under steady-state conditions.

Another property of ligand–receptor interactions is saturability; that is, only a finite number of specific receptor sites exist per unit tissue. This maximum number of specific receptor sites is usually designated as B_{max}.

$$[RL] + [R] = B_{max}$$

multiply by [L]

$$[RL][L] + [R][L] = B_{max}[L]$$

$$[RL][L] + \frac{[RL]}{[RL]}[R][L] = B_{max}[L]$$

substitute Eq. [4] with a = b = c = 1

$$[RL][L] + [RL]K_D) = B_{max}[L]$$

$$[RL]([L] + K_D) = B_{max}[L]$$

$$[RL] = \frac{B_{max}[L]}{[L] + K_D} \qquad [5]$$

which is the classic law of mass action for enzyme–substrate interactions adapted to receptor–ligand interactions (see also Chapter 2). If we now define RL as bound ligand = B, and L as free ligand = F, from Eq. [5]

$$B = \frac{B_{max}F}{F + K_D}$$

$$BF + BK_D = B_{max}F$$

Dividing by F

$$B + \frac{B}{F}K_D = B_{max}$$

transferring fields

$$B/F = \frac{B_{max} - B}{K_D}$$

which is the Scatchard (27) equation. Thus knowing the concentrations of ligand bound and free at equilibrium allows the determination of both the equilibrium binding constant (K_D) and the maximum number of binding sites (B_{max}).

2. *Separating Bound from Free Ligand*

Once the appropriate radiolabeled ligand has been obtained and purified, the investigator must choose an appropriate separation technique. Among other things, the choice of a separation technique depends on whether the receptor under study is in a particulate or a soluble form. For particulate preparations the choice is usually between some form of centrifugation or of filtration. For soluble binding sites, a variety of separation techniques including dialysis, column chromatography, precipitation of receptor–ligand complex, and adsorption of free ligand may be utilized.

The major underlying theoretical constraint on separation techniques is the rate of dissociation of the receptor–ligand complex at the temperature of separation of bound from free ligand. Thus receptor–ligand complexes that dissociate rapidly will require separation techniques that minimize the amount dissociated. Figure 1 shows the relationship between loss of binding due to dissociation of receptor–ligand complex and total separation time (total time that the receptor–ligand complex can dissociate during separation). In Fig. 1 it is assumed that the separation began while the binding reaction was at equilibrium and that the separation time refers to the total time that the receptor–ligand complex is exposed to concentrations of free ligand significantly lower than that present at equilibrium. Figure 1 does not include any correction for reassociation of the ligand to the receptor since with most separation techniques the free ligand concentration is, for all practical purposes, infinitely diluted and the ligand cannot significantly reassociate.

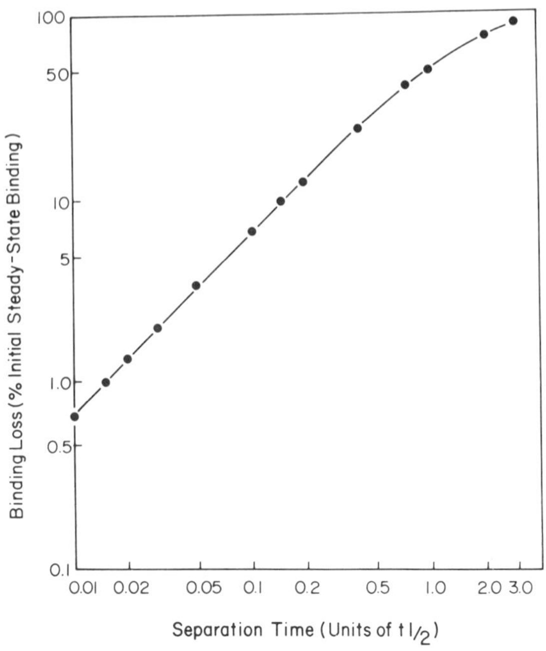

FIG. 1. Loss of receptor–ligand binding due to dissociation of the receptor–ligand complex during separation. Separation time is given in units of half-life (t½) for dissociation of the receptor-ligand complexes. This figure is applicable only to receptor–ligand dissociations which follow first-order kinetics and does not include any correction for reassociation of receptor and ligand.

The loss of binding owing to dissociation increases approximately linearly through the first half-life (Fig. 1). Thus a separation procedure that is complete in less than approximately 0.15 $t_{1/2}$ must be utilized to avoid losing more than approximately 10% of bound ligand. Because it is desirable to wash the receptor–ligand complex as thoroughly as possible to remove free unbound isotope, the time of washing (which is part of the total separation time) plays a crucial role in increasing the total/blank ratio of the procedure.

How much separation time will the actual binding constant (K_D) allow? By assuming that the forward reaction association rate constant is 10^6 M^{-1} sec^{-1} (which is very close to experimentally determined values for most neurotransmitter receptors) one can calculate the following equilibrium relationship:

$$K_D = \frac{k_{\text{dissoc.}}}{k_{\text{assoc.}}} = \frac{0.693/t_{1/2}}{10^6 \text{M}^{-1}\text{s}^{-1}} = \frac{6.93 \times 10^{-7}\text{M} \times \text{sec}}{t_{1/2}}$$

In Fig. 2 K_D is plotted versus the half-life of dissociation in seconds. Since Fig. 1 has revealed that a desirable maximum separation time is approximately 0.15 $t_{1/2}$ to avoid loss of more than 10% bound ligand, approximate upper limits for separation times may be calculated for various equilibrium binding constants (Table 1). Various separation procedures used for ligand-binding studies are discussed below and their respective approximate separation times as well as the relative advantages and disadvantages of each procedure are summarized in Table 2.

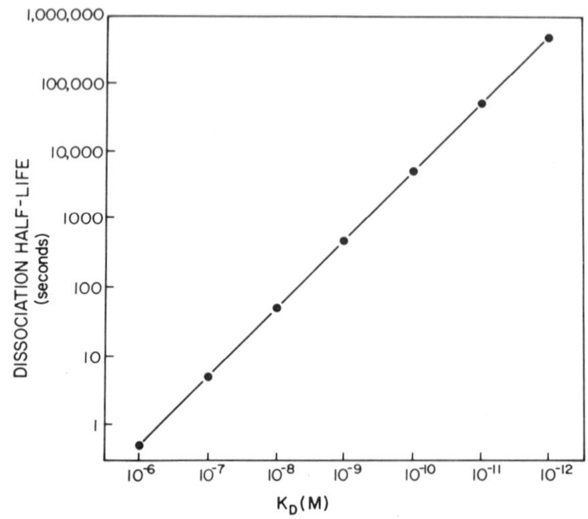

FIG. 2. Relationship between the rate of dissociation of the receptor–ligand complex (presented as the half-life) and the equilibrium dissociation binding constant (K_D). This figure presents hypothetical data for receptor–ligand complexes which obey first-order kinetics during dissociation and associate at the rate of 10^6 M^{-1} × sec.$^{-1}$.

TABLE 1. *Relationship between equilibrium binding constant (K_D) and allowable separation time*

K_D (M)	Allowable separation time (0.15 $t_{1/2}$)[a]
10^{-12}	1.2 days
10^{-11}	2.9 hr
10^{-10}	17 min
10^{-9}	1.7 min
10^{-8}	10 sec
10^{-7}	0.10 sec
10^{-6}	0.01 sec

[a] Calculations of t½ (half-life for dissociation) assume an association rate constant of 10^6 $M^{-1} \times sec^{-1}$.

a. Filtration

Filtration techniques, which are unsurpassed for speed and efficiency, are the most widely used in particulate receptor studies. A most important aspect of filtration is the apparatus used. A well-suited, custom manufactured filtration machine (Fig. 3) has a 45-well manifold in which each 2.5 cm filter is supported by a porous, large mesh, rigid plastic frame. Each filter is then sealed from above by a large bore polyethylene ring. The outside edge of the manifold is seated on a silicone gasket and clamped to a solvent tank underneath. By applying a vacuum to the tank, all filters are subjected to equivalent pressure; individual samples can then be rapidly filtered and the filter wells rapidly rinsed with ice cold buffer. Total elapsed time for filtration and washing (separation time) is on the order of approximately 15 to 20 sec per sample. From Table 1, it is clear that filtration will work only for binding processes with K_Ds of approximately 10^{-8} M or less.

A potential disadvantage of filtration is the nonspecific binding of radioligands to the filter material. A pertinent example of such a phenomenon is the stereospecific binding of radiolabeled opiates to glass fiber filters described by Pasternak and Snyder (24). Thus it is necessary to either select a filter support that minimally binds the radioligand or to include antiadsorbents that minimize this nonspecific binding.

b. Centrifugation

For those particulate receptor–ligand studies with either rapid dissociation of the receptor–ligand complex or in which nonspecific radioligand binding to filter materials cannot be reduced, centrifugation is the best compromise method. The major "compromise" of the centrifugation procedure involves the less efficient washing of the particulate pellet compared to filtration techniques, resulting in higher levels of unbound radioligand trapped in the pellet water space. For

TABLE 2. *Separation procedures for receptor-ligand studies*

Procedure	Separation time: Initial +	Washing =	Total	Advantages	Disadvantages
I. Particulate preparations					
A. Filtration	0[a]	15 sec	15 sec	1. Speed and large sample capacity	1. Nonspecific ligand binding to filter materials
	5–15 sec[b]	15 sec	20–30 sec	2. Most thorough washing (lowest blanks)	2. Limitations as to amount of tissue which can be used without clogging filters
B. Centrifugation					
Macro scale	0[c]	5 sec[d]	5 sec	1. Rapid separation	1. Lower sample number
Micro scale	0[c]	0[e]	0	2. Small volume (micro scale)	2. Less efficient washing (higher blanks)
		10 sec[d]	10 sec		
II. Soluble preparations					
A. Dialysis	0	0	0	1. No separation time-dissociation artifact	1. Limited sample number 2. Nonspecific ligand binding to dialysis membrane
B. Adsorption of free ligand	Min	0	Min	1. Greater sample number than dialysis	1. Long separation time
C. Column chromatography	Min to hr	0	Min to hr	1. Effective for ligands not adsorbable	1. Very long separation time

[a] If incubation homogenate is not diluted before filtering.
[b] If incubation homogenate is diluted with buffer before filtering.
[c] No dilution of incubation homogenate before centrifugation.
[d] Rapid rinsing of pellet and tube.
[e] No washing or rinsing of pellet or tube.

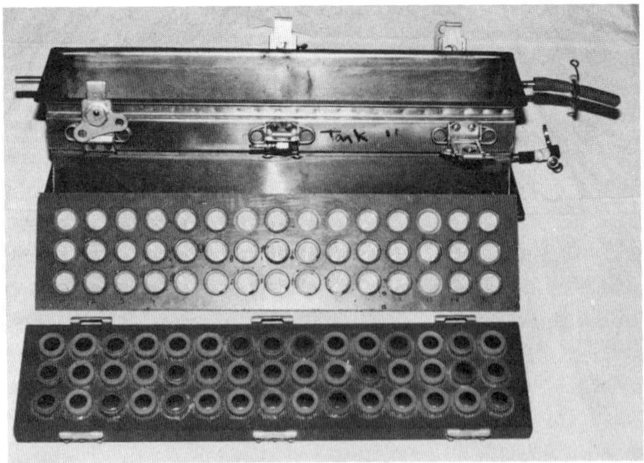

FIG. 3. A 45-well manifold-type filter machine (custom manufactured by E. Sandbeck, Instrument Shop, Johns Hopkins Medical School).

glycine (42) and γ-aminobutyric acid (GABA) (15) synaptic receptors centrifugation procedures are necessary to reproducibly demonstrate receptor binding because of the rapid dissociation rates of [^{3}H]strychnine and [^{3}H]GABA even at 4° C. For other neurotransmitter and hormone receptors, centrifugation procedures give kinetic results comparable to filtration techniques but with higher levels of nonspecific binding owing to sequestered radioligand. Levels of such sequestered radioligand may be reduced by extensive washing of tissue pellets (addition of cold buffer and recentrifugation), but such procedures can become tedious and time consuming and are prohibited in studies of receptor–ligand complexes with rapid dissociation rates.

When conditions necessitate centrifugation, the most critical aspect of the technique involves rapid, careful rinsing of the centrifuge tube and pellet to remove as much unbound radioligand as possible without allowing the rinsing buffer to either remain in contact with the pellet for more than a few seconds, which would result in kinetic (dissociation) loss of receptor–ligand complex, or to disrupt pellet integrity, which would result in mechanical loss of receptor–ligand complex. An interesting modification of centrifugation procedures involves the use of conical microcentrifuge tubes and dibutyl phthalate-dinonyl phthalate oil mixtures (5). When mixed in the ratio of 3:2, the resulting oil is slightly denser than isotonic or hypotonic aqueous buffers but less dense (at room temperature or above) than most brain particulate preparations. Thus a small layer of oil mixture can be placed in the bottom of each microfuge tube and tissue preparation in buffer containing ligands is layered on top. After incubation the samples are centrifuged in microcentrifuges and the tip of the microfuge tube containing the particulate pellet is cut off and bound radioactivity determined. This procedure has the advantage of rapid separation of particulate matter from incubation buffer, but has the disadvantage of inefficient washing of the particulate pellet. Also, very lipophilic radioligands can potentially diffuse into the oil layer, giving elevated and inconsistent "blanks."

c. Equilibrium Dialysis

Dialysis techniques may be used to study both particulate and soluble receptor preparations. Equilibrium dialysis is particularly suitable for receptors with very low affinities for ligands (10^{-7} M or greater) and thus very rapid dissociation rates. Small dialysis cells (less than 1 ml volume) separated by semipermeable membranes allow rapid equilibration of small radioligands between the receptor and buffer sides of the dialysis cell. Equilibrium dialysis has been utilized to measure the saturable binding of cholinergic agonists to solubilized nicotinic cholinergic receptors of invertebrate electric tissues (7) and binding of ^{3}H-LSD to mammalian brain serotonin receptors (16).

The major disadvantage of dialysis techniques involves the small differences in cpm/ml of radioligand usually found between the receptor and the buffer sides of the dialysis membrane. If less than 10% of added ligand is bound, then the receptor side of the dialysis membrane would contain at most approximately 20% more cpm/ml than the buffer side. Because of the low affinities of receptors usually studied by dialysis, large amounts of receptor protein must be added to one side of the dialysis chamber to achieve significant binding. For purified receptor proteins such as the invertebrate nicotinic cholinergic receptor, this problem is surmountable because of the very high degree to which this receptor has been purified. In addition it is necessary to determine if the dialysis membrane contributes significantly to radioligand binding. No low-affinity mammalian neurotransmitter receptors have, to date, been studied by equilibrium dialysis (the K_D for ^{3}H-LSD binding is in the nanomolar range).

d. Gel Filtration Chromatography

For solubilized or physiologically soluble receptor preparations, gel filtration provides a sensitive but tedious method for detection of bound radioligand. The gel filtration procedure may be performed in one of two general ways. First, a receptor and a ligand are incubated to equilibrium and applied to an appropriate resin bed preequilibrated with incubation buffer. In the course of column elution (which can take hours) receptor-bound ligand is separated from free ligand and quantitated. The second procedure is based on the technique originally developed by Hummel and Dreyer (20) and discussed quantitatively by Cuatrecasas et al. (13). The resin bed is equilibrated with elution buffer containing a small concentration of radioligand. Receptor preparation is then applied to the top of the column and elution is carried out with more eluting buffer containing radioligand. Receptor-bound radioligand appears as a "peak" of radioactivity above baseline and is followed by a "trough" of radioactivity; bound ligand can then be calculated knowing the radioactivity present in the "peak" and "trough" (13,20).

Such gel filtration techniques have been utilized extensively in studies of cytoplasmic steroid hormone receptors in mammalian brain and other tissues (19). As might be predicted, the major limiting constraint is the dissociation rate of the receptor–ligand complex as it passes through the column. In addition, the resin bed offers the possibility of nonspecific binding of radioligand, a condition that must be ruled out.

e. Precipitation of Receptor–Ligand Complex and Adsorption of Free Ligand Techniques

Both of these techniques have been utilized in studies of soluble hormone receptors. Because of the limited number of studies performed on solubilized neurotransmitter receptors, these techniques are presented primarily for purposes of potential application.

The precipitation technique depends on the decreased solubility of large proteins on addition of structural perturbing agents such as ammonium sulfate, salting out agents, acid, or polyethylene glycol. Success with the precipitation technique depends on the rapidity with which the receptor–ligand complex can be precipitated with respect to the ligand dissociation rate, and the dissociation rate of ligand from precipitated complex compared to the speed with which the precipitated complex can be isolated. Successful receptor–ligand studies using the precipitation technique include those of solubilized insulin (10) and nicotinic cholinergic (22) receptors.

The adsorption of free ligand technique, widely used in radioimmunoassay procedures, utilizes the selected adsorption of unbound radioligand to a slurry of inert support (e.g., talc, charcoal). Frequently the inert support can be coated with a carbohydrate polymer (Dextran) to incorporate a molecular sieving action that increases the selectivity of the procedure. Small unbound molecules rapidly penetrate the Dextran "shell" and are bound by the inert support whereas large receptor–ligand complexes are excluded from access to the adsorbent. The adsorbent is isolated by centrifugation or filtration and unbound ligand is determined. The difference between total radioligand present and unbound ligand adsorbed to the support represents macromolecularly bound ligand, but potential nonspecific radioligand binding to test tubes, filters, and so forth, must be assessed. If centrifugation is used to pellet the adsorbent, then the major limitation of the procedure is that the dissociation rate of the ligand from the receptor–ligand complex (in the supernatant) must have a half-life of at least seven times the total separation time to avoid significant (greater than 10%) loss of bound ligand.

3. The Experimental Blank

Radiolabeled chemicals used as ligands in receptor-binding studies possess remarkable abilities to bind nonspecifically to both biological and nonbiological substances. Hollenberg and Cuatrecasas (11) found that radiolabeled insulin could bind to talc with affinities in the nanomolar range, not too far from the affinity of insulin for its biological receptor. This radiolabeled insulin binding also exhibited apparent negative cooperativity, a phenomenon that has been described for true biological receptor–ligand interactions. Thus care and caution are needed in establishing the criteria for nonspecific binding in a receptor–ligand assay.

Several criteria have been utilized, depending on the particular receptor–ligand studied, to establish nonspecific binding. In general, specific binding is taken as the difference between total binding and binding that occurs in the presence of an excess concentration of unlabeled ligand (100 times K_D concentration). Note that under these conditions the nonspecific ligand binding may be composed of several components: (a) true nonspecific binding to the tissue under study, (b) free radioligand not effectively washed away, and (c) nonspecific binding to separation materials (filters, test tubes, etc.). Very rarely can true tissue nonspecific binding be reduced. However, it is necessary to determine experimentally if the washing procedure is as effective as possible by comparing different numbers of washes, volumes of washing buffers, and so forth. Significant nonspecific radioligand binding to separation materials, if present, can frequently be reduced by including antiadsorbents in the assay system. Examples of such antiadsorbents are albumin or collagen for radioiodinated peptides and o-catechol for tritiated catecholamine-binding studies (2,37–39). It is essential to ensure that the antiadsorbent added does not in itself bind significant amounts of the radioligand, thus reducing the available free ligand concentration. The well characterized ability of serum albumin to bind many drugs serves as an example of how an antiadsorbent can potentially interfere with the binding assay. Practically, as low a concentration of antiadsorbent as possible should be used to lower nonspecific binding. To check for interference by the antiadsorbent in the binding assay, saturation experiments can be performed in the presence of increasing concentrations of the antiadsorbent. If significant alterations in the apparent binding constant are observed with increasing concentrations of antiadsorbent, then it may be reasonably assumed that the antiadsorbent is itself binding the radioligand to a significant extent and an appropriate concentration of antiadsorbent can be chosen or a different antiadsorbent tried.

Many central nervous system receptors such as the muscarinic cholinergic, and α- and β-nonadrenergic receptors have homogolous receptors in the periphery that have been well characterized pharmacologically. For such well characterized receptors many drugs with structures markedly different from that of the radioligand used to bind to the receptor interact potently at the receptor site, and an excess concentration of any of these unlabeled drugs can be used to determine nonspecific radioligand binding. When possible, it is always best to use a displacing ligand that is chemically different from the radioligand to increase the probability of obtaining receptor-specific binding. Examples of this methodology are outlined in Table 5.

4. Metabolism of the Radioligand

In all radioligand-binding studies it is obligatory to demonstrate that radioligands both bound to the receptor and free in solution are not metabolized or degraded. A complete study of potential ligand metabolism should include analysis of both bound and free radioligand by conventional analytical procedures (i.e., TLC, electrophoresis) and also by rebinding studies. The conventional assay techniques are familiar to most; suffice it to say that at least two different systems should be utilized and that the migration of radioligand (after exposure to the tissue receptor should be compared to migration of radioligand) not exposed to receptor but cospotted with homologous tissue extract.

Rebinding studies provide very sensitive evidence about metabolism or degradation of radioligands. The basic procedure is that bound ligand is eluted off receptor sites, usually under mild acidic or denaturing conditions, and is rebound to a fresh receptor preparation alongside fresh, previously unexposed radioligand. The fresh and exposed radioligands are added to the receptor preparation in equal concentrations (cpm/ml). After this rebinding study, the binding of exposed and previously unexposed radioligand is compared in terms of (a) the percent of total added cpm that is bound, (b) the ratios of total/blank and specific/blank binding. At equal cpm/ml concentrations of exposed and unexposed radioligands, these two results should be equal if no metabolism or structural alterations have taken place. In addition, the original unbound (free) radioligand should be examined by rebinding studies as well.

From past experience it is known that the ligands most likely to be degraded in central nervous system receptor studies are natural products or derivatives of natural products for which brain tissue possesses catabolic pathways (i.e., catecholamines, peptides). Overcoming this catabolism usually involves inhibition of the catabolic enzymes by including various drugs such as MAO or peptidase inhibitors. In certain instances it is necessary to reduce the incubation temperature of the binding study to eliminate detectable ligand catabolism.

For substances susceptible to nonenzymatic oxidative degradation (e.g., catecholamines, D-LSD) or light (e.g., dihydromorphine) it will be necessary to add antioxidants or incubate in the dark to overcome these possible forms of degradation.

III. ANALYSIS OF BINDING DATA

A. Saturation Experiments

1. Scatchard Plots

Determination of the equilibrium binding constant and apparent maximum number of binding sites for a given radioligand and tissue receptor involves incubating various concentrations of the radioligand with a fixed concentration of tissue, measuring the amount of ligand bound, and analyzing the data according to the Scatchard equation as previously presented in this chapter. The concentration of the radioligand may be increased in one of two ways. One way is to increase the amount of radioligand added and keep the specific activity of the radioligand constant, thereby increasing cpm in the incubation volume. A second method is to hold the concentration of radioactivity constant in the incubation medium and increase the concentration of unlabeled ligand, thus in effect increasing the ligand concentration by diluting the specific activity of the radioligand. Both of these techniques have inherent advantages and disadvantages, and in a complete saturation study both techniques should be utilized as the data generated are complementary. Before attempting a ligand saturation study, the previously discussed criteria of radioligand purity, possible radioligand metabolism, and minimization of nonspecific binding must be satisfied. In addition, tissue linearity of radioligand binding with respect to the tissue of interest should have been demonstrated and the appropriate incubation time and temperature to reach a steady state determined. Ideally all radioligand-binding studies should be performed in "zone A" such that at equilibrium less than 10% of the added radioligand is bound to the tissue (35). This is important because the investigator must know the actual concentration of free ligand present at steady state in order to calculate the binding constant. If zone A conditions are maintained then a loss of up to 10% of added radioligand concentration will not significantly affect the estimation of binding constants when it is assumed that the added radioligand concentration is equal to actual free radioligand concentration at equilibrium. If, however, greater than 10% of added radioligand is bound at equilibrium, then serious underestimations of the actual binding constant will occur unless the investigator takes into account the actual free ligand concentration at steady state.

With these precautions in mind it is best to proceed in initial experiments by using as small a concentration of radioligand as is possible to reliably measure ligand binding in the tissue under investigation and obtain an estimate of the binding constant by then adding increasing amounts of unlabeled ligand to generate a ligand displacement curve. Assuming that the unlabeled ligand behaves at the receptor site very similarly to the labeled ligand (which may not be the case) and that binding phenomena under investigation follow classic mass action, then the concentration of unlabeled ligand at which the maximum binding of labeled ligand is displaced by 50% (IC_{50}) will be a reasonable first approximation of the apparent equilibrium dissociation binding constant (K_D). Once this first estimate is obtained, the investigator should compare this estimated K_D to the actual concentration of radioligand present in this initial binding study. As a general rule, the concentration of radioligand present should be at least one-fourth or less than that of the concentration of unlabeled ligand giving 50% displacement. As the concentration of radioligand [L] utilized in displacement studies is increased, the difference between the IC_{50} of unlabeled

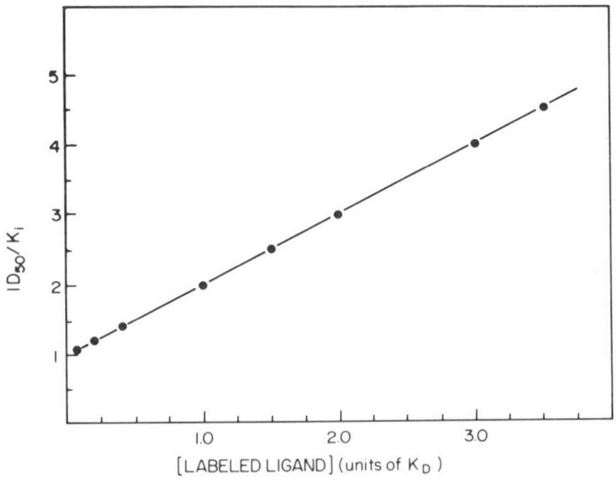

FIG. 4. Relationship between the concentration of radioligand used in a binding study, the K_D of the radioligand for the binding site, the concentration of unlabeled ligand giving half-maximal displacement (IC_{50}) of radioligand, and the affinity constant for binding of the unlabeled ligand to the same binding site (K_i). The data presented indicate that as the concentration of radioligand in a binding assay increases, the deviation of the IC_{50} for an unlabeled compound from the true K_i of the unlabeled compound progressively increases. This is applicable only to binding studies where the radioligand and unlabeled compound interact competitively at the binding site.

ligand and the binding affinity constant of unlabeled ligand (K_i) progressively widens at fixed tissue concentration according to the following equation, which is also represented graphically in Fig. 4 (8):

$$K_i = \frac{IC_{50}}{1 + [L]/K_D}$$

It should be noted that this equation applies only to binding phenomena where labeled and unlabeled ligand interact competitively at the receptor site.

The concentration of receptor sites in the incubation medium can also influence the relationship between IC_{50} and true K_i. Jacobs et al. (21) point out that the relationship among IC_{50}, K_i, K_D, and receptor site concentration at steady state is

$$IC_{50} = n(K_D + L_t + R_t - 3/2RL) = K_i + n(L_t + R_t - 3/2RL)^*$$

where L_t and R_t refer to the total concentrations of radiolabeled ligand and receptor sites, respectively, RL refers to concentration of receptor–radioligand complex formed in the absence of unlabeled ligand, and $K_i = nK_D$. If $(L_t + R_t) \ll K_d$, then the IC_{50} will approximate the K_i. In practice, the concentration of total receptor sites should thus not exceed approximately 10% of the

* Adapted from Eq. 10 in ref. 21.

K_D for a given radioligand when estimating affinity constants by competitive displacement.

Once this initial estimate of the K_D is obtained by a displacement study, it is possible to proceed to a more detailed estimate of the K_D using radioligand saturation studies. In these studies, the concentration of radioactivity is increased in the incubation medium while the specific activity of the radioligand is held constant. The amount of radioligand specifically bound at each radioligand concentration is then determined, radioligand bound is converted to moles of radioligand bound per unit weight of tissue or tissue protein and fitted into the Scatchard equation. An example of such a study that is taken from actual experimental data is presented in Table 3. In this study of mammalian brain serotonin receptors, increasing concentrations of tritiated serotonin ([^{3}H]5-HT) were incubated with rat hippocampal membranes at 37°C for 10 min utilizing a buffer system that had previously been shown to protect [^{3}H]5-HT from catabolism (1). The initial estimate of the binding constant for [^{3}H]5-HT under these conditions was found to be about 8 nM; thus, the 5-HT binding was evaluated over a concentration range of approximately one-sixth the estimated K_D to approximately four times the estimated K_D. In Table 3, all steps in the analysis of the data are presented beginning with "raw" data of cpm added, cpm bound (specific) and leading through the conversion of these data to pmoles of [^{3}H]5-HT bound per gram of tissue, and analysis of these according to the Scatchard equation. The actual data presented in terms of a Scatchard plot are shown in Fig. 5. Conventional linear regression techniques may be used to calculate the line or lines of best fit. After the best fit for the data is obtained the equilibrium dissociation constant (K_D) is estimated as the negative reciprocal of the slope of the line of best fit, and the apparent maximum number of binding sites (B_{max}) is estimated by the abscissa intercept of the line. The major advantage of the Scatchard equation compared to other methods of plotting saturation data is that all points in the graph are given equal statistical weight. The experimental error in determining the major variable, bound radioligand, is mathematically eliminated from the line fitting procedure because the variable is present on both axes.

2. *Hill Plots*

The majority of neurotransmitter receptor–ligand interactions studies to date have followed classic mass action laws, at least with respect to any single radioligand's binding in saturation studies or displacement by the structurally identical unlabeled compound (32). However, in many neurotransmitter–receptor-binding studies, displacement of a given radioligand from its receptor by unlabeled compounds different from the radioligand has yielded anomalous behavior, most commonly apparent as negatively cooperative interactions (Hill plot slope significantly less than one). These situations have arisen primarily in instances of a radiolabeled antagonist being displaced by an unlabeled agonist or vice-versa.

TABLE 3. [^{3}H]5-HT *binding saturation to rat hippocampal membranes*[a]

Scatchard plot data

[^{3}H]5-HT added		[^{3}H]5-HT bound (cpm)			[^{3}H]5-HT bound/free	
cpm/2 ml × 10^{-4}	nM[b]	Total −	Blank =	Specific	pmol/g tissue[c]	pmol/g-nM × 10
4.06	1.21	1,358	321	1,037	3.24	26.8
8.12	2.41	2,208	541	1,667	5.21	21.6
12.2	3.62	3,097	719	2,378	7.43	20.5
16.2	4.83	3,910	1,041	2,869	8.96	18.6
24.4	7.24	5,294	1,524	3,770	11.8	16.3
61.0	18.1	9,665	4,358	5,306	16.6	9.17
122	36.2	15,843	9,148	6,695	20.9	5.77

Hill plot data

[^{3}H]5-HT (nM)	log	$\frac{B}{(\text{pmol/g})}$	$\frac{B}{B_{max}-B}$	$\log \frac{B}{(B_{max}-B)}$
1.21	0.083	3.24	0.146[d]	−0.836[d]
2.41	0.382	5.21	0.258	−0.588
3.62	0.559	3.43	0.413	−0.384
4.83	0.684	8.96	0.546	−0.263
7.24	0.860	11.8	0.868	−0.0616
18.1	1.26	16.6	1.89	0.276
3.62	1.56	20.9	4.64	0.667

[a] [^{3}H]5-HT (16.2 Ci/mmol) was incubated with 2 ml aliquots of rat hippocampal membranes containing 20 mg wet weight of tissue per sample. Blank samples represent binding in the presence of 10^{-5} M unlabeled 5-HT. Particulate-bound [^{3}H]5-HT trapped on glass filters was counted at 44% efficiency.

[b] Because less than 3% of added [^{3}H]5-HT was bound, total added [^{3}H]5-HT is set equal to "free" [^{3}H]5-HT in these calculations.

[c] $\frac{\text{cpm specific [}^3\text{H]5-HT}}{44\%\ \text{efficiency}} \times \frac{1\ \text{nCi}}{2.24 \times 10^3\ \text{dpm}} \times \frac{1\ \text{pmol[}^3\text{H]5-HT}}{16.2\ \text{nCi}} \times \frac{1}{0.02\ \text{g tissue}}$.

[d] These data are calculated using a B_{max} of 25.4 pmol/g determined from the Scatchard plot (Fig. 5).

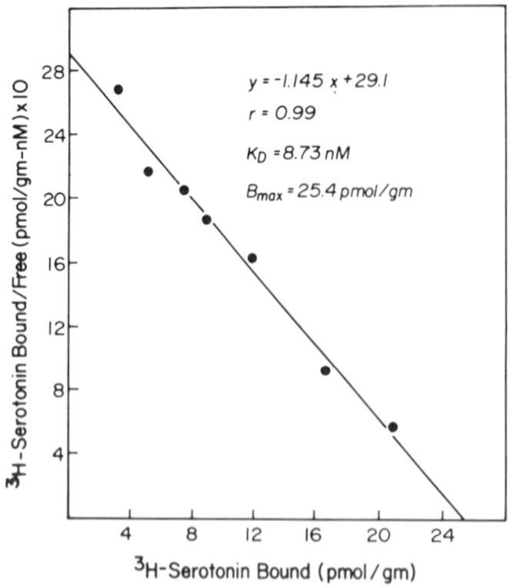

FIG. 5. Scatchard plot of the binding of [^{3}H]5-HT to rat hippocampal membranes. The data for construction of the Scatchard plot are presented in Table 3.

Such findings have prompted theoretical considerations of kinetically separable but interacting agonist–antagonist-binding sites of a given neurotransmitter receptor (32). Regardless of the interpretation of the findings, the important point for this discussion is the use of Hill plots to detect and "quantitate" such anomalous behavior. Thus in this section Hill plots will be presented from the standpoint of derivation of the Hill equation and practical application to binding studies. Theoretical considerations of interpreting Hill plots will not be discussed; the reader is referred to separate reviews of this subject (12,30).

The Hill equation was derived to quantitate the deviations of enzyme–substrate interactions from classic mass-action, rectangular hyperbolic behavior. One of the earliest applications of the Hill equation was to the oxygen saturation of hemoglobin, where it is known that binding of the first O_2 molecule facilitates the binding of the second O_2 molecule and so forth. Instead of obeying classic mass action law

$$B = \frac{B_{max}[\text{Ligand}]}{K_D + [\text{Ligand}]}$$

such systems could be adapted to a sequential ligand-binding model

$$R + L \overset{K_{D_1}}{\rightleftharpoons} (R - L)_1$$

$$(R - L)_1 + L \overset{K_{D_2}}{\rightleftharpoons} (R - L)_2$$

$$(R - L)_2 + L \overset{K_{D_3}}{\rightleftharpoons} (R - L)_3$$

$$\ldots\ldots (R - L)_{n-1} + L \overset{K_{D_n}}{\rightleftharpoons} (R - L)_n$$

with

$$B = \frac{B_{max}[\text{Ligand}]^n}{K_D' + [\text{Ligand}]^n} \qquad [6]$$

describing the net ligand-binding isotherm. In this model n = theoretical number of ligand-binding sites per receptor molecule, K_D' = a composite constant composed of the intrinsic dissociation constant (K_D) and interaction factors that determine the degree to which K_D is altered at each discrete binding step.

Rearranging Eq. [6] yields

$$\frac{B}{B_{max}} = \frac{[L]^n}{K_D' + [L]^n}$$

which is the Hill equation.

The Hill equation may be transformed to a logarithmic form for convenience in plotting as follows:

$$B_{max}[L]^n = B\,K_D' + B[L]^n$$

$$\frac{[L]^n(B_{max} - B)}{B} = K_D'$$

$$n\log[L] + \log\frac{(B_{max} - B)}{B} = \log K_D'$$

$$\log\frac{(B_{max} - B)}{B} = \log K_D' - n\log[L]$$

or

$$\log\frac{B}{(B_{max} - B)} = n\log[L] - \log K_D' \qquad [7]$$

Fitting ligand-binding data into Eq. [7] is straightforward and may be performed using either saturation or displacement experiments. An example of fitting saturation data into the Hill equation (logarithmic form) is presented in the second half of Table 3. The saturable binding of [^{3}H]5-HT to rat hippocampal membranes was first fitted into the Scatchard equation and plotted (Fig. 5). The Scatchard plot yielded a B_{max} of 25.4 pmol/g which was used in fitting the saturation data to the Hill equation (Table 3). The data are plotted in Fig. 6. The points all fit on a straight line with a slope of 0.94, which is so close to unity that the Hill number (n_H) can be considered equal to one.

Thus in this example the ligand binding obeys classic mass actions laws because the Hill equation

$$\frac{B}{B_{max}} = \frac{[L]^n}{K_D' + [L]^n}$$

reduces to

$$B = \frac{B_{max}[L]}{K_D' + [L]}$$

when n = 1.

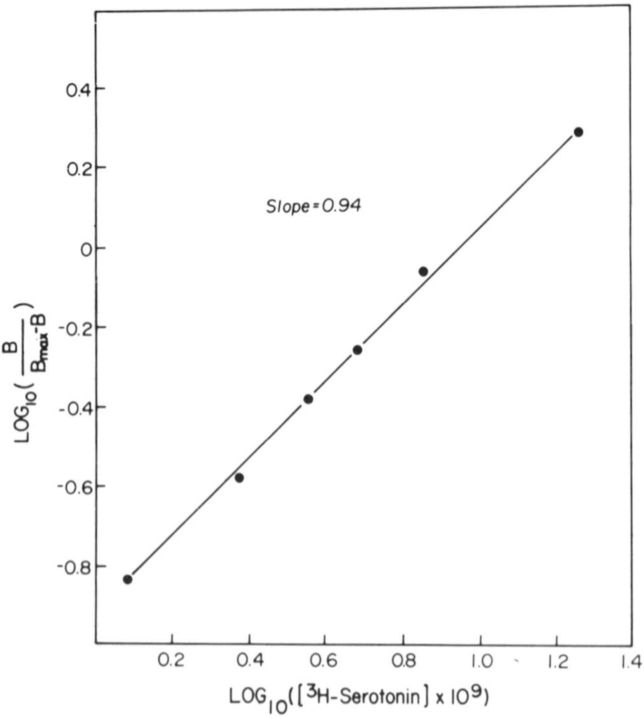

FIG. 6. Hill plot of [^{3}H]5-HT binding to rat hippocampal membranes. The data are derived in the lower half of Table 3.

The Hill binding constant, K_D', is calculated as the abscissa value where log $[B/(B_{max} - B)] = 0$. In Fig. 6, the K_D' is thus antilog $(0.97) \times 10^{-9} = 9.3$ nM, a value not significantly different from the K_D determined by Scatchard analysis (8.7 nM).

In displacement experiments where a fixed concentration of radiolabeled ligand is incubated with increasing concentrations of unlabeled ligands, the resulting data may also be analyzed by Hill plots. In this case, the specific radioligand binding (total minus blank) occurring in the absence of any displacing agents is taken as B_{max}. Binding occurring in the presence of displacing agents can be expressed as percentage of B_{max}. The data can then be plotted as log $[\%B_{max}/(100\% - \%B_{max})]$ versus log [displacer] to yield the Hill plot.

B. Rate Constants

As previously discussed, the equilibrium binding constant is a ratio of the binding reaction's forward and reverse rate constants. For this reason, it is desirable to estimate the rate constants for association (k_a) and dissociation (k_d) so that the binding constant derived from saturation data may be compared to the binding constant resulting from the ratio of rate constants. In most ligand–receptor studies, the binding constants derived by these two independent means are equal within experimental error.

This discussion will be limited to the most basic of reaction models, that is, bimolecular association

$$R + L \rightarrow RL$$

which follows second-order kinetics, and unimolecular dissociation

$$RL \rightarrow R + L$$

which follows first-order kinetics. For all neurotransmitter receptors studied to date, the binding constants calculated from such a model are equal, within error, to the binding constants derived from equilibrium saturation studies.

1. Association Rate Constant

The simple rate equation for bimolecular association

$$\frac{d[RL]}{dt} = k_a[R][L] \qquad [8]$$

when integrated yields

$$k_a = \frac{2.303}{t[L - R]}\left(\log\frac{R[L - x]}{L[R - x]}\right) \qquad [9]$$

with R and L equal to the unoccupied receptor and free ligand, respectively, at time t_o, and x equal to the amount of each consumed in time t. Theoretically, Eq. [9] will enable the calculation of k_a for any bimolecular binding reaction when R, L, and x are known. However, for binding studies performed with 10% or less of the total available ligand bound by equilibrium, k_a estimated from Eq. [9] will be subject to large error because x will never exceed 10% of L. This problem is further compounded because experimentally it is desirable to measure initial ligand association rates where ligand–receptor dissociation causes minimal error on estimation of k_a. Thus in practice it is not unusual to estimate k_a based on data where 5% at most of initial free ligand is bound to receptor.

More theoretically and experimentally practical methods to estimate k_a should be used. One such technique is to perform the binding experiment under pseudo-first-order conditions with respect to both free ligand and unoccupied receptor. If an initial free ligand concentration one-half of the K_D or less for that ligand is used and binding data only up through the first half-life of association are analyzed, then, at most, only approximately one-eighth of the total receptor sites will be occupied and [R] can be assumed equal to $B_{max} \times$ [tissue]. Likewise, if tissue concentration is controlled so as to be in zone A behavior (35), then [L] does not change appreciably and can also be considered constant. Eq. [8] then reduces to

$$\frac{d[RL]}{dt} = k_a'$$

where $k_a' = k_a[R][L]$

$$d[RL] = k_a' dt \quad [10]$$

To estimate k_a, specifically bound ligand is plotted versus time. The best line of fit through, at most, the first half-life is constructed; the slope of this line, k_a' is then divided by the initial concentrations of free ligand ([L]) and receptor ([R] = $B_{max} \times$ [tissue]) to yield k_a.

The second method takes into consideration the contribution of ligand–receptor dissociation to the eventual reaching of a steady state. Bound ligand is assayed at various time intervals up to the steady-state level (B_{eq}). $Ln[B_{eq}/(B_{eq} - B_t)]$ is plotted versus time where B_t is the amount of specifically bound ligand at time t. The slope of this line (k_{obs}) is related to the association (k_1) and dissociation (k_{-1}) rate constants, and free ligand concentration, [L], as follows:

$$k_1 = \frac{k_{obs} - k_{-1}^*}{[L]} \quad [11]$$

This equation is valid only when the binding reaction is performed with no more than 10% of initial free ligand bound at steady state. Estimating k_1 by this method requires knowledge of the dissociation rate constant (k_1) as described in the next section.

2. Dissociation Rate Constant

The dissociation rate constant (k_{-1}) is estimated by incubating radioligand and receptor for a given period of time, usually to steady state, and then "infinitely" diluting the radioligand concentration. After various time intervals specifically bound radioligand is then measured. The half-life ($t_{1/2}$) for loss of specifically bound radioligand is determined from a plot of log [RL] versus time, and k_{-1} is calculated as $0.693/t\frac{1}{2}$. Alternatively, the slope of log [RL] versus time multiplied by −2.303 yields k_{-1}.

"Infinite" dilution of radioligand may conveniently be done two different ways which are complementary to each other. Ideally, both methods should be utilized to search for contributions of cooperativity to the binding process, as discussed below. In the first method, a concentrated solution of receptor and ligand is incubated to steady state and then diluted with at least a 100-fold volume excess of incubation buffer at the temperature of the dissociation study. Aliquots of "infinitely" diluted receptor–ligand mixture are assayed for bound radioligand at various time intervals afterward. In the second method, receptor preparation and radioligand are incubated to steady state and a 1,000-

* For derivation see Appendix A.

fold molar excess of unlabeled ligand is added. Thus as each radioligand molecule dissociates from its receptor, the odds of an unlabeled ligand molecule reassociating in its place are 1,000 times greater than before addition of unlabeled ligand. Receptor-bound radioligand is assayed at various time intervals thereafter.

By performing dissociation studies using both of these methods, it is possible to determine if the presence of excess unlabeled ligand accelerates the dissociation rate compared to volumetric "infinite" dilution. If excess unlabeled ligand accelerates the dissociation rate, then negative cooperativity may be a part of the binding process. Apparent negative cooperativity in dissociation studies may also arise artifactually at higher receptor and low ligand concentrations due to the "retention effect." (31) As the receptor site concentration approaches or exceeds the K_D of the radioligand, diffusion of dissociated radioligand away from free receptor sites is progressively hampered, probably because of the very high local concentrations of unoccupied binding sites. In other words, radioligand reassociation rate (k_a [R] [L]) becomes fast enough to compete with radioligand diffusion rate (α[L]) away from binding sites. The retention effect could influence estimation of dissociation rate constants by volumetric "infinite" dilution but not by adding excess unlabeled ligand. Should excess unlabeled ligand accelerate radioligand dissociation compared to volumetric "infinite" dilution, the volumetric dilution experiments should be performed at several final tissue concentrations to rule out possible contributions of retention effect.

C. Potential Artifacts in Receptor Studies

Many of the potential artifacts of receptor–ligand-binding studies have previously been discussed in this chapter. The major sources of artifacts may conveniently be categorized as belonging primarily to the ligand, the tissue under study, or the separation procedure utilized. In Table 4, potential problems in receptor–ligand-binding studies arising from each of these three sources are discussed, the artifacts generated by each one of these problems are delineated, and suggestions are given for methods of detection of the artifacts.

IV. INDIVIDUAL NEUROTRANSMITTER RECEPTORS

The purpose of this section is to give a detailed overview of the various radioligands and methods available to study synaptic receptor sites for compounds that are fairly well "established" as neurotransmitters in the mammalian central nervous system. Because many of the mechanical procedures for the various neurotransmitter receptor-binding studies are similar, the details can conveniently be presented in tabular form (Table 5). The details so presented are taken from the literature and represent many conditions found essential to optimize each individual ligand's binding. However, many of the details have some degree of flexibility, such as tissue preparation, and thus may be modified by the individual investigator.

TABLE 4. *Potential artifacts in receptor-binding studies*

Source	Problem	Artifact(s)	Detection
I. Ligand	Radiochemical purity, specific activity	Overestimation of true ligand concentration with underestimation of binding constant or vice versa	1. Quantitative and qualitative analysis of radiochemical purity 2. Disparate binding parameters by saturation compared to displacement
	Self-association	Apparent negative cooperative behavior in dissociation studies (excess unlabeled ligand accelerates dissociation rate compared to infinite dilution); Such behavior may indicate the presence of true negative cooperative behavior as well	Use displacing agents (in dissociation studies) structurally different from ligand
	Association to antiadsorbent	Alteration of experimental K_D	Saturation studies with different concentrations of antiadsorbent, if utilized
	Different affinities of labeled vs. unlabeled ligand	Nonlinear Scatchard plots, apparent cooperative behavior	Comparison of Scatchard and Hill plots using labeled ligand alone and labeled ligand displaced by unlabeled ligand
II. Tissue	Nonreceptor saturable ligand binding	Apparent receptors	Structure activity studies
	Ligand metabolism	Binding of ligand metabolites, overestimation of free ligand concentration	Metabolism studies
	Tissue concentration too high (greater than 10% of added ligand bound)	Underestimation of binding constant	Knowledge of true free ligand concentration at equilibrium
III. Separation procedure	Separation procedure too slow for ligand dissociation rate	Loss of binding, underestimation of B_{max}, inaccurate determination of K_D	Comparison of K_D determined by equilibrium compared to kinetic studies
	Ligand binding to separation materials	Excessively high blanks, possible additional "receptor" populations	Ligand binding in absence of tissue

V. SUMMARY

Radiolabeled neurotransmitter agonists and/or antagonists can be used as ligands in binding studies to characterize ligand recognition sites of neurotransmitter receptors. Success in ligand-binding studies depends on many factors involving the radioligand, methods for separating bound from free ligand, and proper analysis of binding data. The two most commonly utilized isotopes for ligand radiolabeling are tritium and, where appropriate, ^{125}I. Investigators must always be cognizant of the radioligand's purity, specific activity, biological activity, proper storage, potential metabolism, and nonspecific binding.

The major theoretical constraint in assessing various receptor-bound ligand separation procedures is the dissociation rate of the receptor–ligand complex. Some separation procedures are thus limited in application because of the time they allow for receptor–ligand dissociation. In addition, the separation procedure, as well as every other variable in ligand-binding studies, may lead to experimental artifacts.

Saturable, steady-state binding data is best analyzed by Scatchard plots that allow equal statistical weight to be applied to all points. Hill plots may be constructed to search for evidence of cooperative interactions. Estimations of association and dissociation rate constants are straightforward once the underlying kinetic principles are understood.

Finally, a detailed overview of currently available neurotransmitter–receptor binding procedures is presented.

VI. APPENDIX A: DERIVATION OF INTEGRATED EQUATION FOR ASSOCIATION RATE CONSTANT

Abbreviations: L = unbound ligand; R = unoccupied receptor; RL = receptor–ligand complex.

$$\mathrm{L} + \mathrm{R} \underset{k_{-1}}{\overset{\mathrm{k}_1}{\rightleftharpoons}} \mathrm{RL} \qquad [1]$$

defines the general second order association and first order dissociation binding processes. The association rate equation is

$$\frac{\mathrm{d[RL]}}{\mathrm{dt}} = k_1[\mathrm{L}][\mathrm{R}] - k_{-1}[\mathrm{RL}] \qquad [2]$$

If the binding experiment is performed in zone A (35), [L] remains essentially constant and a new association rate constant k_1' can be defined as $k_1' = k_1[\mathrm{L}]$. Substituting into Eq. [2] yields

$$\frac{\mathrm{d[RL]}}{\mathrm{dt}} = k_1'[\mathrm{R}] - k_{-1}[\mathrm{RL}] \qquad [3]$$

TABLE 5. *Neurotransmitter receptor procedures—part A*

Neurotransmitter	Source	Tissue preparation[a]	Tissue concentration (mg protein/ml)	Incubation: Buffer[b]	Incubation: Temp. (°C)	Incubation: Time (min)	Radioligand
1. Acetylcholine	Mammalian CNS	1	0.2–0.4	A	25	60	[^{3}H]Quinuclidinyl benzilate (QNB)
2. γ-Aminobutyric acid (GABA)	Mammalian CNS	1–3	0.4–0.6	B	4	5	[^{3}H]GABA
3. Dopamine	Mammalian caudate	1	0.5–1.0	C	37	10	[^{3}H]Dopamine (DA)
				C	37	10	[^{3}H]Haloperidol (HALO)
				C	37	10	[^{3}H]Spiroperidol (SPIRO)
				D	22	30	[^{3}H]Apomorphine (APO)
4. Glycine	Mammalian CNS	2	0.5	E	4	10	[^{3}H]Strychnine (STRY)
5. α-Noradrenergic	Mammalian CNS	1	1.0	F	25	45 (in the dark)	[^{3}H]Dihydroergokryptine (DHE)
				G	37	5	[^{3}H](−)-Norepinephrine (NE)
				H	37	5	[^{3}H](−)-Epinephrine (EPI)
6. β-Noradrenergic	Mammalian CNS	1	0.5	I	23	20	[^{3}H]Dihydroalprenolol (DHA)
	Mammalian CNS	4	0.5	J+ 0.1 mm phentolamine, 1 mm Na ascorbate	37	18–30	[^{125}I]Hydroxybenzylpindolol (HYP)
	Chick CNS	2	1–2	K	23	15	[^{3}H]DL-4*n*-Propranolol (PROP)
	Calf cerebellar cortex	1	1.0	G+ 1 μM Pargyline	4	30	[^{3}H]EPI
7. Serotonin	Mammalian CNS	1	0.5–1.0	L	37	10	[^{3}H]D-Lysergic acid diethylamide (LSD)
	Mammalian CNS	1	0.5–1.0	L	37	10	[^{3}H]5-HT

[a] Tissue preparation procedures:

1. Total particulate pellet. Tissue is disrupted in 20 to 40 volumes of ice cold buffer (eg. F) using a mechanical homogenizer such as the Polytron. Total particulate material is isolated by centrifugation (4°C) at high speed, commonly 50,000 × *g* for 5 to 10 min. The pellet is washed one or more times by rehomogenization in buffer and recentrifugation and then suspended in appropriate incubation buffer.
2. Crude synaptic membrane (CSM) pellet. Fresh (not previously frozen) tissue is homogenized in 10 to 20 volumes of ice cold 0.32 M sucrose using a close-fitting Teflon pestle in a glass tube (Potter-Elvehjm). The crude nuclear pellet (P1) is isolated by centrifugation (4°C) at 1,000 × *g* for 10 min and discarded. The supernatant is centrifuged at 17,000 × *g* for 10 min to yield the crude mitochondrial pellet (P2). P2 is lysed by homogenization in at least 10 volumes of ice cold H_2O and centrifuged at 8,000 × *g* for 20 min. The supernatant and soft upper "buffy coat" of the pellet are collected and centrifuged at 50,000 × *g* for 10 min to yield the CSM pellet. For both glycine and GABA receptor studies, the CSM should be frozen before use, then washed with cold H_2O before resuspension in incubation buffer.
3. CSM pellet-Triton X-100 treated. The CSM pellet is resuspended in buffer B to a protein concentration of about 1 mg/ml (approximately 100 volumes of original tissue weight). Triton X-100 is added to a final concentration of 0.05% (v/v) and the homogenate incubated at 37°C for 30 min. The treated CSM fraction is isolated by centrifugation (50,000 × *g* for 10 min) and resuspended in buffer B for receptor assay.
4. The unlysed P2 pellet (see item 2, above) is resuspended in 70 volumes of buffer J.

[b] Incubation buffers:

A. 50 mM Na-K phosphate, pH 7.4.
B. 50 mM Tris-citric acid, pH 7.1 at 4°C.
C. 50 mM Tris-HCl with 0.1% ascorbic acid, 10 μM pargyline, 120 mM NaCl, 5 mM KCl, 2 mM $CaCl_2$, and 1 mM $MgCl_2$ with final pH 7.1 at 37°C.
D. 15 mM Tris-HCl (pH 7.4 at 22°C) with 5 mM Na_2EDTA, 1.1 mM ascorbic acid, and 12.5 μM nialamide.
E. 50 mM Na-K phosphate (pH 7.1) with 200 mM NaCl.
F. 50 mM Tris-HCl, pH 7.7 at 25°C.
G. Buffer F with 0.003% ascorbic acid, 1 mM pyrocatechol, 0.1 mM Na_2EDTA, and 10 μM dithiothreitol.
H. Same as buffer G except 50 mM Tris-HCl (pH 8.0 at 25°C) is used.
I. 50 mM Tris-HCl (pH 8.0 at 25°C) with 0.1% ascorbic acid and 1 μM pargyline.
J. 0.9% NaCl with 20 mM Tris-HCl (pH 7.5 at 37°C).
K. 50 mM Tris-HCl with 15 mM $MgCl_2$ (pH 8.1 at room temperature).
L. 50 mM Tris-HCl with 0.1% ascorbic acid and 10 μM pargyline (pH 7.2 at 37°C).

TABLE 5. *Neurotransmitter receptor procedures—Part B*

Radioligand					
Name	Source	Concentration (nM)	Blank	Separation/wash[a]	Ref.
[^{3}H]QNB	Commercial	0.1	1 μM Atropine 0.1 mM Oxotremorine	Filtration—GF/B; 3 × 3 ml wash with buffer A (4°C)	41
[^{3}H]GABA	Commercial	8	0.1 mM Bicuculline 1 mM GABA	Centrifugation at 4°C. 2 × 5 ml rinses with buffer B (4°C)	15
[^{3}H]DA	Commercial	5	1 μM DA 10 μM (+)Butaclamol	Filtration—GF/B. 2 × 5 ml wash with buffer F (4°C)	3
[^{3}H]HALO	Commercial	2	0.1 mM DA 0.1 μM (+)Butaclamol	Same as above	3
[^{3}H]SPIRO	Commercial	0.2	1 mM DA 1 μM (+)Butaclamol	Same as above	28
[^{3}H]APO	Catalytic exchange tritiation	1.5–3.3	1 μM (+)Butaclamol	Filtration—GF/B. 2 × 5 ml wash with buffer D (23°C)	29
[^{3}H]STRY	Catalytic exchange tritiation	2	0.1 mM Strychnine	Centrifugation at 4°C. 2 × 5 ml rinses with buffer E (4°C)	42
[^{3}H]DHE	Commercial	0.3–0.4	1 mM (−)NE	Filtration—GF/B. 2 × 5 ml wash with buffer F (4°C)	17
[^{3}H](−)NE α-adrenergic	Commercial	2	10 μM (−)NE 0.1 μM Oxymetazoline	Filtration—GF/B presoaked in buffer F with l mM pyrocatechol. 2 × 5 ml wash with buffer F (4°C) containing 1 mM pyrocatechol and 0.1% ascorbic acid	38
[^{3}H](−)EPI (α-adrenergic)	Commercial	5	10 μM (−)NE 0.1 μM Oxymetazoline	Filtration—GF/B presoaked in buffer F with 1 mM pyrocatechol. 2 × 5 ml wash with buffer F (4°C) containing 1 mM pyrocatechol and 0.1% ascorbic acid	38
[^{3}H]DHA	Commercial	1	1 μM (−)Alprenolol	Filtration—GF/B. 3 × 5 ml wash with buffer F (4°C)	4

[^{125}I]HYP	Iodination	0.03	0.3 μM (±)Propranolol	Addition of 10 ml buffer I (37°C) 45 sec later, filtration Gelman A-E, 1 × 10 ml wash with buffer J	33
[^{3}H]PROP	Commercial	15	0.2 mM (−)Isoproterenol	Filtration—GF/C. 1 × 10 ml wash with buffer K	23
[^{3}H](−)EPI (β-adrenergic)	Commercial	10	0.1 μM (±)EPI 1 μM (±)Propranolol	Same as for H-(−)NE and ^{3}H-(−)EPI in α-adrenergic	39
[^{3}H]LSD	Commercial	3	1 μM d-LSD 0.1mM 5-HT	Filtration—GF/B. 2 × 5 ml wash with buffer F (4°C)	1
[^{3}H]5-HT	Commercial	7	10 μM 5-HT 0.1 mM d-LSD	Same as above	1

[a] Separation/wash procedures:

1. Filtration—incubation samples are rapidly filtered under vacuum in an apparatus such as that in Fig. 2. The incubation tubes and filter wells are washed with indicated amounts of buffer. GF/B and GF/C refer to Whatman glass-fiber filters.
2. Centrifugation—incubation samples are centrifuged (4°C) at high speed (50,000 × *g*) for 5 min. Supernatants are discarded and the pellets and inside tube walls rapidly and carefully rinsed with ice cold buffer. The tubes are allowed to drain, and the inside tube walls are carefully wiped free of excess buffer. A small amount (1 ml) of tissue solubilizer (e.g., Protosol®) is added to solubilize the radioactivity.

At any given time t the concentration of unoccupied receptor ([R]) is equal to

$$[\mathrm{R}] = [\mathrm{R}]_o - [\mathrm{RL}]_t \qquad [4]$$

At equilibrium, the net formation of RL is zero. Substituting Eq. [4] into Eq. [3] at equilibrium yields

$$k_1'([\mathrm{R}]_o - [\mathrm{RL}]_{eq}) = k_{-1}[\mathrm{RL}]_{eq} \qquad [5]$$

$$k_{-1} = \frac{k_1'[\mathrm{R}]_o}{[\mathrm{RL}]_{eq}} - k_1' \qquad [6]$$

Substituting Eq. [6] into Eq. [3]

$$\frac{\mathrm{d}[\mathrm{RL}]}{\mathrm{dt}} = k_1'([\mathrm{R}]_o - [\mathrm{RL}]) - \left(\frac{k_1'[\mathrm{R}]_o}{[\mathrm{RL}]_{eq}} - k_1'\right)[\mathrm{RL}] \qquad [7]$$

Eq. [7] reduces to

$$\frac{\mathrm{d}[\mathrm{RL}]}{\mathrm{dt}} = k_1' \frac{[\mathrm{R}]_o([\mathrm{RL}]_{eq} - [\mathrm{RL}])}{[\mathrm{RL}]_{eq}} \qquad [8]$$

which rearranges to

$$\frac{\mathrm{d}[\mathrm{RL}]}{[\mathrm{RL}]_{eq} - [\mathrm{RL}]} = \frac{k_1[\mathrm{R}]_o}{[\mathrm{RL}]_{eq}}\,\mathrm{dt} \qquad [9]$$

Integrating Eq. [9] from t_1 to t_2 yields

$$\ln\frac{[\mathrm{RL}]_{eq} - [\mathrm{RL}]_{t_1}}{[\mathrm{RL}]_{eq} - [\mathrm{RL}]_{t_2}} = \frac{k_1'[\mathrm{R}]_o}{[\mathrm{RL}]_{eq}}(t_2 - t_1) \qquad [10]$$

Eq. [10] is a general equation that can be used for any two time points on the association curve for an equilibrium process. Eq. [10] can be further reduced by setting $t_1 = 0$; therefore $[\mathrm{RL}]_{t_1} = 0$.

$$\ln\frac{[\mathrm{RL}]_{eq} - 0}{[\mathrm{RL}]_{eq} - [\mathrm{RL}]_{t_2}} = \frac{k_1'[\mathrm{R}]_o\, t_2}{[\mathrm{RL}]_{eq}} \qquad [11]$$

From Eq. [6]

$$k_{-1} + k_1' = \frac{k_1'[\mathrm{R}]_o}{[\mathrm{RL}]_{eq}} \qquad [12]$$

Substituting Eq. [12] and $k_1' = k_1[\mathrm{L}]$ into Eq. [11] yields

$$\ln\frac{[\mathrm{RL}]_{eq}}{[\mathrm{RL}]_{eq} - [\mathrm{RL}]_t} = (k_{-1} + k_1[\mathrm{L}])\,t \qquad [13]$$

A plot of $\ln\frac{[\mathrm{RL}]_{eq}}{[\mathrm{RL}]_{eq} - [\mathrm{RL}]_t}$ versus time yields a line with a slope

$$k_{obs} = k_{-1} + k_1[\mathrm{L}]$$

Therefore

$$k_1 = \frac{k_{obs} - k_{-1}}{[L]}$$

ACKNOWLEDGMENTS

I would like to thank Dr. David C. U'Prichard for helpful discussions concerning the theoretical aspects of certain derivations presented in this chapter and acknowledge support by USPHS Fellowship DA-05055.

VII. REFERENCES

1. Bennett, J. P., Jr., and Snyder, S. H. (1976): Serotonin and lysergic acid diethylamide binding in rat brain membranes: Relationship to postsynaptic serotonin receptors. *Mol. Pharmacol.,* 12:373–389.
2. Bennett, J. P., Jr., and Snyder, S. H. (1976): Angiotensin II binding to mammalian brain membranes. *J. Biol. Chem.,* 251:7423–7430.
3. Burt, D. R., Creese, I., and Snyder, S. H. (1976): Properties of [^{3}H] haloperidol and [^{3}H] dopamine binding associated with dopamine receptors in calf brain membranes. *Mol. Pharmacol.,* 12:800–812.
4. Bylund, D. B., and Snyder, S. H. (1976): Beta adrenergic receptor binding in membrane preparations from mammalian brain. *Mol. Pharmacol.,* 12:568–580.
5. Chang, K-J., and Cuatrecasas, P. (1974): ATP-dependent inhibition of insulin-stimulated glucose transport in fat cells—possible role of membrane phosphorylation. *J. Biol. Chem.,* 249:3170–3180.
6. Changeux, J. P., Kasai, M., and Lee, C. Y. (1970): Use of a snake venom toxin to characterize the cholinergic receptor protein. *Proc. Natl. Acad. Sci. USA,* 67:1241–1247.
7. Changeux, J. P., Meunier, J-C., and Hughet, M. (1971): Studies on the cholinergic receptor protein of Electrophorus electricus. 1. An assay in vitro for the cholinergic receptor site and solubilization of receptor protein from electric tissue. *Mol. Pharmacol.,* 7:538–553.
8. Cheng, Y-C., and Prusoff, W. H. (1973): Relationship between the inhibition constant (K_i) and the concentration of inhibitor which causes 50 percent inhibition (I_{50}) of an enzymatic reaction. *Biochem. Pharmacol.,* 22:3099–3108.
9. Cuatrecasas, P. (1971): Insulin-receptor interaction in adipose tissue cells: Direct measurement and properties. *Proc. Natl. Acad. Sci. USA,* 68:1264–1268.
10. Cuatrecasas, P. (1972): Isolation of the insulin receptor of liver and fat cell membranes. *Proc. Natl. Acad. Sci. USA,* 69:318–322.
11. Cuatrecasas, P., and Hollenberg, M. D. (1975): Binding of insulin and other hormones to non-receptor materials: Saturability, specificity, and apparent "negative cooperativity." *Biochem. Biophys. Res. Commun.,* 62:31–41.
12. Cuatrecasas, P., and Hollenberg, M. D. (1976): Membrane receptors and hormone action. *Adv. Protein Chem.,* 30:251–451.
13. Cuatrecasas, P., Fuchs, S., and Anfinsen, C. B. (1967): Catalytic properties and specificity of the extracellular nuclease of Staphylocus aureus. *J. Biol. Chem.,* 242:3063–3067.
14. Eldefrawi, M. E., Britten, A. G., and Eldefrawi, A. T. (1971): Acetylcholine binding to torpedo electroplax: Relationship to acetylcholine receptor. *Science,* 173:338–340.
15. Enna, S. J., and Snyder, S. H. (1977): Influences of ions, enzymes, and detergents on γ-aminobutyric acid-receptor binding in synaptic membranes of rat brain. *Mol. Pharmacol.,* 13:442–453.
16. Farrow, J. T., and Van Vunakis, H. (1972): Binding of D-lysergic acid diethylamide to subcellular fractions from rat brain. *Nature (Lond),* 237:164–166.
17. Greenberg, D. A., and Snyder, S. H. (1977): Selective labeling of α-noradrenergic receptors in rat brain with [^{3}H]dihydroergokryptine. *Life Sci.,* 20:927–932.
18. Greenwood, F. C., and Hunter, W. M. (1963): The preparation of ^{131}I-labelled human growth hormone of high specific activity. *Biochem J.,* 89:114–123.

19. Grosser, B. I., Stevens, W., and Reed, D. J. (1973): Properties of corticosterone-binding macromolecules from rat brain cytosol. *Brain Res.,* 57:387–395.
20. Hummel, J. P., and Dreyer, W. J. (1962): Measurement of protein-binding phenomena by gel filtration. *Biochim. Biophys. Acta,* 63:530–532.
21. Jacobs, S., Chang, K-J. and Cuatrecasas, P. (1975): Estimation of hormone receptor affinity by competitive displacement of labeled ligand; Effect of concentration of receptor and of labeled ligand. *Biochem. Biophys. Res. Commun.,* 66:687–692.
22. Munier, J-C., Sealock, R., Olsen, R., and Changeux, J-P. (1974): Purification and properties of the cholinergic receptor protein from Electrophorus electricus electric tissue. *Eur. J. Biochem.,* 45:371–394.
23. Nahorski, S. R. (1976): Association of high affinity stereospecific binding of [^{3}H]propranolol to cerebral membranes with β-adrenoceptors. *Nature (Lond),* 259:488–489.
24. Pasternak, G. W., and Snyder, S. H. (1975): In: *Neurosciences Research Program Bulletin, Vol. 13: Opiate Receptor Mechanisms,* edited by S. H. Snyder and S. Matthysse, p. 27. Neurosci. Res. Prog., MIT Press, Boston.
25. Pataki, G. (1966): *Techniques of Thin-Layer Chromatography in Amino Acid and Peptide Chemistry.* de Gruyter, Berlin.
26. Raftery, M. A., Schmidt, J., and Clark, D. G. (1972): Specificity of α-bungarotoxin binding to Torpedo california electroplax. *Arch. Biochem. Biophys.,* 152:882–926.
27. Scatchard, G. (1949): The attractions of proteins for small molecules and ions. *Ann. NY Acad. Sci.,* 51:660–672.
28. Schneider, R., Creese, I., and Snyder, S. H. (1978): ^{3}H-Spiroperidol labels pituitary and brain dopamine receptors. *Eur. J. Pharmacol. (in press).*
29. Seeman, P., Lee, T., Chau-Wong, M., Tedesco, J., and Wong, K. (1976): Dopamine receptors in human and calf brains, using [^{3}H] apomorphine and an antipsychotic drug. *Proc. Natl. Acad. Sci. USA,* 73:4354–4358.
30. Segel, I. H. (1975): *Enzyme Kinetics,* pp. 360–373. Wiley-Interscience, New York.
31. Silhavy, T. J., Szmelcman, S., Boos, W., and Schwartz, M. (1975): On the significance of the retention of ligand by protein. *Proc. Natl. Acad. Sci. USA,* 72:2120–2124.
32. Snyder, S. H., and Bennett, J. P., Jr. (1976): Neurotransmitter receptors in the brain: Biochemical identification. *Annu. Rev. Physiol.,* 38:153–175.
33. Sporn, J. R., and Molinoff, P. B. (1976): β-Adrenergic receptors in rat brain. *J. Cyclic Nucleotide Res.,* 2:149–161.
34. Stahl, E., editor (1969): *Thin-Layer Chromatography: A Laboratory Handbook.* Springer-Verlag, New York.
35. Straus, O. H., and Goldstein, A. (1943): Zone behavior of enzymes. *J. Gen. Physiol.,* 26:559.
36. Thorell, J. I., and Johansson, B. G. (1971): Enzymatic iodination of polypeptides with ^{125}I to high specific activity. *Biochim. Biophys. Acta,* 251:363–369.
37. Uhl, G. R., Bennett, J. P., Jr., and Snyder, S. H. (1977): Neurotensin, a central nervous system peptide: Apparent receptor binding in brain membranes. *Brain Res.,* 130:299–313.
38. U'Prichard, D. C., and Snyder, S. H. (1977): [^{3}H]Epinephrine and [^{3}H]norepinephrine binding to α-noradrenergic receptors in calf brain membranes. *Life Sci.,* 20:527–534.
39. U'Prichard, D., and Snyder, S. H. (1977: Differential labeling of α and β noradrenergic receptors in calf cerebellum with ^{3}H-adrenaline. *Nature (Lond),* 270:261–263.
40. Werman, R. (1972): CNS cellular level membranes. *Annu. Rev. Physiol.,* 34:337–374.
41. Yamamura, H. I., and Snyder, S. H. (1974): Muscarinic cholinergic binding in rat brain. *Proc. Natl. Acad Sci. USA,* 71:1725–1729.
42. Young, A. B., and Snyder, S. H. (1973): Strychnine binding associated with glycine receptors of the central nervous system. *Proc. Natl. Acad. Sci. USA,* 70:2832–2836.

Neurotransmitter Receptor Binding, edited by
H. I. Yamamura et al.
Raven Press, New York © 1978.

5

Biochemical Studies of Receptors: Solubilization, Purification, Characterization, and Studies with Antibodies

Jon M. Lindstrom

The Salk Institute, San Diego, California 92112

I. INTRODUCTION

A. Problems in Biochemical Studies of Receptors

Biochemical studies of receptors are usually directed at answering two types of questions: (a) What molecular structures are responsible for the ligand-binding properties of the receptor? and (b) What molecular mechanisms are involved in transducing the binding of a neurotransmitter to its receptor into a physiologically relevant signal? A neurotransmitter receptor is usually thought of in terms of an integral membrane protein (61)[1] with an enzyme-like active site for ligand binding whose occupancy by an agonist induces a conformational change in the protein that regulates an ion channel in the membrane (3), or a nucleotide cyclase (46), or some other signal amplifying device that may or may not be an integral part of the receptor macromolecule. In the case of the nicotinic acetylcholine receptor, experiments (21) suggest that the latency between acetylcholine binding and increase in membrane conductance occurs on a scale of microseconds, and that the ion channel probably closes as the acetylcholine molecule dissociates, approximately a millesecond later. This suggests that the ligand binding and effector components of the acetylcholine receptor are probably intimately associated in a single macromolecular complex. On the other hand, the β-adrenergic receptor appears to exist as an independent unit that can be transferred from one adenylate cyclase system to another. This was elegantly demonstrated by Orly and Schramm (46), who fused cells having functional receptors with cells having functional cyclase to produce conjugates that exhibited adrenergically regulated cyclase activity. Several receptors of the same or differing specificity can share the same effector when rapidity of signal transmission is not at issue.

Four types of problems usually beset biochemical studies of receptors. Probably the most important is the vanishingly small amount of receptor available in most tissues. Thus purification of many of the neurotransmitter receptors in brain might be expected to require development of a procedure beginning with kilograms of tissue, achieving purification by factors of many thousands, and yielding finally only micrograms of protein for further study. The second barrier to biochemical studies is solubilizing the receptor from membranes and then identifying it in the extracts. The third problem is developing a purification method that can achieve adequate concentration, purification, and yield of receptor from the extract. The fourth, and thus far most difficult problem, is reconstitution of the purified receptor into an artificial membrane so that it retains its signal transducing function. This is really in part a problem of purification, because until the purified receptor can be shown to be both homogeneous and to retain all the functional properties it possessed *in situ* without deletion or denaturation, purification is not complete. An entirely different approach to purification may be required to obtain a homogeneous preparation of native receptor than that which may be used to obtain a homogeneous but denatured preparation.

B. The Acetylcholine Receptor as an Example

The problems besetting purification of receptors have been surmounted with varying degrees of success depending on the receptor involved. Progress has

[1] Referencing throughout this chapter is not exhaustive, with, in many cases, review articles cited rather than primary references.

been greatest in the case of the nicotinic acetylcholine receptor. Because this receptor is the best characterized neurotransmitter receptor both physiologically and biochemically, it can be hoped that it may provide something of an archetype for the study of other receptors.

In the case of the acetylcholine receptor, the problem of low concentration in muscle [e.g., 1.1×10^{-12} mol/g human leg muscle (30)] was solved by finding a richer source in the form of fish electric organs [e.g., 1×10^{-9} mol/g *Torpedo californica* electric organ (54)]. Another fortuitous gift of nature helped solve the problem of identifying the receptor in tissue extracts. Certain snake venom toxins, for example, toxin III of cobra venom or α-bungarotoxin from krait venom, bind with great affinity and specificity to acetylcholine receptors (26). Because these small [8,000 molecular weight (mw)] toxins were proteins, they could easily be labeled to high specific activity with ^{125}I. Binding specificity in intact tissue was established both by inhibition of ^{125}I-toxin binding to the tissue by appropriate agonists and antagonists (3,54) and by autoradiographic localization of bound ^{125}I-toxin in the endplate zone of normal muscle and extrajunctional regions of denervated muscle (27). Specific binding of ^{125}I-toxin was proportional to inhibition of receptor activity (32). Thus when detergent extracts of electric organ (42) and muscle (1) were shown to contain appropriate amounts of a toxin-binding component that sedimented on sucrose gradients as a single symmetric peak, it was quite reasonable to believe that this macromolecule composed part or all of the physiologically significant receptor. Receptor was still a minor component even of electric organs, and purification of a detergent-solubilized membrane protein made the problem even more complex. Affinity chromatography (4) provided an easy solution to purification. Binding specificity of receptor was, after all, its best characterized feature. Affinity adsorbents for solubilized receptor were prepared using synthetic acetylcholine analogs (54), and even more easily and specifically by using cobra venom toxin (32). In a single step, receptor was specifically adsorbed from crude detergent extracts and rigorously washed free of unbound contaminants. Synthetic ligand columns bind both acetylcholine esterase and acetylcholine receptor. The two proteins are separately eluted using a gradient of increasing salt concentration (54). Cobra toxin columns specifically bind only receptor and are eluted by competition with a cholinergic ligand, giving a second step of affinity purification. Because the history of ligand binding to the acetylcholine receptor affects its ligand-binding affinity (3), and because its conformation would be expected to be altered by the transition from postsynaptic membrane to detergent micelle, it was not surprising to discover that the ligand-binding specificity of the purified receptor differed somewhat from that in intact membrane (3). It was pleasantly surprising that the acetylcholine binding site survived at all. But what of the ion channel regulated by acetylcholine binding? Was it hopelessly denatured, or not part of the toxin-binding macromolecule, or perhaps never solubilized from the membrane in the first place? Reconstitution of purified acetylcholine receptor into an artificial membrane in such a way that it can be rigorously and reproducibly shown that the appropriate ligands produce the appropriate conductance changes across the membrane has not, despite many claims, been demonstrated. Only when this step has been achieved will it be demonstrable that the complete and intact functional receptor macromolecule has been purified. A reconstituted system could then provide an excellent model for beginning studies of the molecular biology of receptor function.

Fortunately, yet another gift of nature has given us something to do while we wait for reconstitution to work. Animals immunized with purified acetylcholine receptor develop an autoimmune response to their skeletal muscle nicotinic acetylcholine receptors (48). This has proven a remarkably useful model for investigating pathologic mechanisms in a human disease, myasthenia gravis, subsequently shown also to involve an autoimmune response to receptor (30). The antibodies that mediate the autoimmune response are useful reagents because they are directed at determinants on the receptor molecule other than the binding site for cholinergic ligands. They can be used to provide an easy radioimmune assay for solubilized receptor. Antibodies can, at least in principle, provide templates for comparison of specific, defined structures in purified electric organ receptor with structures of unpurified or even membrane-bound receptor from muscle. Antibodies can inhibit receptor function (15,51). And antibodies can affect receptor metabolism by increasing turnover (15).

In the following sections the problems in purification of receptors will be considered, often with reference to the acetylcholine receptor. I will largely ignore the problem of the small amounts of receptors available, except to suggest that using primary cultures or cloned cells may have certain advantages. The amounts of receptor obtainable may be smaller than can usually be obtained from, for example, brain, but the amount of other receptors and extraneous material to remove during purification may be a lot less. More importantly, the function of a receptor in a cultured cell can be readily assayed (49). As a result, it is more probable that the method used for labeling receptor during purification is associated with a functionally significant receptor, as opposed to simply a ligand binding site of unknown function purified from a detergent extract of homogenized brain. Also, the question of identifying the physiologically significant site by ligand binding will be largely ignored because that is considered elsewhere in this book. Instead, the following sections will be confined to brief comments on solubilization, purification, and characterization techniques.

II. SOLUBILIZATION

A. Methods

Integral membrane proteins such as the acetylcholine receptor in skeletal muscle and electric organ tissue interact through hydrophobic interactions with the lipid bilayer that surrounds them (61). The acetylcholine receptor is strongly negatively charged at neutral pH (3,19,54) and has substantial amounts of carbohydrate associated with all of its component polypeptide chains (3,19,54), presumably, like other membrane proteins that span the lipid bilayer (61), on the extracellular surface of the molecule. These features should make it quite hydrophilic, and its overall amino acid composition (3,19,54) is not remarkably hydrophobic. Thus, presumably, the hydrophobic residues in its component polypeptide chains are arrayed on the interior of the protein and at the periphery which interacts with the hydrophobic interior of the lipid bilayer. To solubilize such an integral membrane protein it is necessary to replace its hydrophobic interactions with the interior of the membrane with hydrophobic interactions with detergent molecules. Some detergents solubilize receptor very efficiently. For example, a 1-min exposure to 1% Triton X-100 will quantitatively solubilize acetylcholine receptors from the plasma membrane of cultured muscle cells and leave the intact-appearing cells complete with nuclei and striations sitting in the dish (6). The solubilized receptors retain their capacity to specifically bind toxins and cholinergic ligands. On the other hand, 1% sodium dodecyl sulfate will solubilize most proteins and denature them to uniform rod-shaped detergent–polypeptide chain aggregates (64).

Detergents vary widely in molecular structure, but share the common feature of having both hydrophilic and hydrophobic regions. Hydrophilic regions may contain charged residues, as in the case of dodecyl sulfate or cholate, or the hydrophilic region may be nonionic like the polyoxyethylene groups of the Triton or Tween detergents. The hydrophobic region may consist of long hydrocarbon chains as in dodecyl sulfate, Triton, and Tween, or of the hydrophobic side of a rigid cyclophenanthrene ring structure as in cholate and deoxycholate. In aqueous solution detergents through hydrophobic interactions form aggregates termed micelles. The size, shape, and stability of the micelles depend on detergent structure, ionic strength, temperature, and other factors. Detergents as dissimilar in structure and properties as Triton X-100 and sodium cholate are both capable of solubilizing the acetylcholine receptor in conformations capable of specifically binding toxin and cholinergic ligands. Ligand-binding properties of the acetylcholine receptor change on solubilization (3). It is still too early in these studies to determine which detergent, if either, solubilizes the receptor in a conformation that closely resembles the native receptor. Thus when first embarking on the solubilization of a receptor, the choice of detergent is usually made empirically and quite pragmatically depending on convenience. For example, although cholate is somewhat less effective at solubilizing acetylcholine receptors than Triton X-100, it has the advantage over Triton X-100 in that it forms small micelles that are readily removed by dialysis and in that it does not absorb at 280 mμ, and so does not interfere with monitoring protein concentration by absorbance at 280 mμ. Excellent reviews (16,64) on the properties of detergents useful for solubilizing proteins are available.

Receptors need not necessarily be solubilized to be purified. The sodium pump from kidney is purified by selective cholate extraction of the purified membranes to remove unwanted proteins (22). In this case, addition of Triton X-100 yields a molecularly disperse protein, but its function is impaired. In the postsynaptic membrane, acetylcholine receptors are packed in dense arrays (3,19,54) and are the principal protein components of the membrane. It has been possible by differential centrifugation and isopycnic density gradient centrifugation to purify membrane vesicles that are 50% receptor (3,19,54,63). In some cases the receptor is still active, and carbamylcholine-induced increase in sodium conductance can be demonstrated *in vitro* (20).

Integral membrane proteins can also be solubilized by agents like 3 M KSCN, urea, guanidine hydrochloride, or succinylation. But these are severe denaturing conditions. Glycophorin, an archetypic membrane protein of the erythrocyte membrane, is extracted using lithium diiodosalicylate (40). This is a severe denaturing condition and seems to work because of the high carbohydrate content of this protein. Tryptic cleavage alone solubilizes the extracellular carbohydrate-rich portion of glycophorin, leaving the C-terminal portion of the polypeptide chain in the membrane (39). Neurotransmitter receptors that are required to possess the subtlety to transduce the tiny energies involved in transmitter binding into some other signal are unlikely to tolerate this sort of brutalization with their function intact.

Peripheral membrane proteins are associated with the surface of the membrane. Acetylcholinesterase monomers are aggregated into groups resembling bunches of grapes (55) on a collagen-like vine (38) attached to the basement membrane. Acetylcholinesterase can be solubilized by high ionic strength (1 M NaCl) or by collagenase. Although this may be a good way to anchor a protein that functions in the intersynaptic space, it is unlikely that neurotransmitter receptors involved both in binding a ligand on the external surface and transducing this signal to the cell could accomplish their function from a peripheral localization. However, a water soluble acetylcholine-binding protein has been isolated from housefly brains (43). Whether this is an acetylcholine receptor, and whether it functions like those in muscle, remains to be determined.

B. Identification of Solubilized Receptors

Measurement of ligand-binding activity of solubilized receptor depends largely on the method previously used to label the receptor *in situ.* Affinity labeling a receptor *in situ* eliminates the problem of labeling it after solubilization. Affinity labeling reagents consist of two functional regions (60); one confers affinity for the receptor site, and the other is capable of reacting covalently with an amino acid side chain in the site. In theory, high-affinity binding of the reagent to the site so greatly enhances the rate of covalent reaction with an appropriately located reactive group in the receptor site that the amount of the reagent reacting in the site is significant with respect to the total amount of reagent bound at all other reactive groups in the preparation. Affinity labeling of the acetylcholine receptor has been achieved (18). This method has several advantages. Because the labeling is covalent, the specificity of labeling can be established *in situ* when the receptor is still functional, and denaturing detergents such as sodium dodecyl sulfate can be used for solubilization. Also, the polypeptide chain marked with the radioactive labeling reagent can be identified by electrophoresis in sodium dodecyl sulfate on acrylamide gels, immediately providing information about the molecular weight of the chain or chains contributing to the ligand-binding site of the receptor molecule. Unfortunately, there are also several disadvantages to affinity labeling. Design and synthesis of an effective affinity labeling reagent is difficult, and depends a great deal on serendipity. Use of photoaffinity labeling reagents (56) can, in principle, eliminate some of the serendipity. Photoaffinity labeling reagents contain a group that is activated by UV light. After UV activation, the group becomes so reactive that it can insert in carbon–hydrogen bonds, with the result that no especially reactive residue has to be located in correct orientation in the binding site. Photoaffinity labeling reagents also have the advantage that in the dark, before they are activated by UV irradiation, they can be used reversibly. Photoaffinity labeling derivatives of proteins (67) and polypeptide hormones (5) have been prepared by relatively simple methods that might be applicable to peptide neurotransmitters. The biggest disadvantage of affinity labeling is that, even with the best of reagents and preparations (18), its specificity has barely proved adequate to identify neurotransmitter receptors. Only 10 to 20% of the labeling reagent bound to eel electric organ tissue is specifically bound to acetylcholine receptor (18). For this reason, affinity labeling reagents may prove most valuable in characterizing already purified receptors (17), where the demands for labeling specificity are much lower. Another drawback of affinity labeling reagents is that they irreversibly inactivate the receptor, prohibiting assay of its function, and prohibiting its purification by affinity chromatography.

Equilibrium dialysis can be used to detect the binding of readily reversible ligands (43). However, the method is slow and laborious, and requires that the binding macromolecule be present at concentrations comparable to the K_D for binding. Receptor at such concentrations is likely to be had in only special cases such as extracts of electric organ tissue.

Very high-affinity ligands that are very slowly reversible and that are highly specific are the ideal. Snake neurotoxins with specificity for the acetylcholine receptor (27) are the perfect examples. Toxin can remain bound to receptors present in low concentration, so that a toxin labeled component can be readily identified by chromatography or sucrose gradient centrifugation. Toxins bound to macromolecules can be separated from unbound toxin by ammonium sulfate or polyethylene glycol precipitation of the bound complex. The small positively charged toxin bound to the large negatively charged acetylcholine receptor can be readily assayed by adsorbing this complex to DEAE filter paper, which does not bind the free toxin (57). Naturally occurring (30) antibodies to receptor or antibodies prepared to the purified component (51) can be used in several ways to provide a simple, rapid, and quantitative radioimmunoassay for solubilized receptor.

III. PURIFICATION

A. Affinity Chromatography

Methods employed for purification of receptors must overcome at least three types of problems: (a) low amounts of receptor, (b) low concentration of receptor and high concentrations of extraneous material, and (c) the presence of detergent that may obscure differences in bulk properties of solubilized proteins. Conventional methods for protein purification separate molecules according to size, shape, and density (e.g., gel filtration chromatography or centrifugation on sucrose gradients) or according to charge (e.g., salting out, ion exchange chromatography, electrophoresis, or isoelectric focusing). It is difficult to apply many of these techniques to large volumes containing a trace component. Because the degree of resolution of most of these techniques is relatively low, several steps depending on different features of the protein to be purified must be combined, and yield decreases at each step.

For purification of neurotransmitter receptors, affinity chromatography is by far the most desirable method. Affinity chromatography achieves purification according to the specific ligand-binding properties of the protein to be purified. The ligand-binding properties of a solubilized neurotransmitter receptor are most likely its best characterized biochemical features. The method of affinity chromatography consists of using a specific ligand conjugated to an insoluble support (such as an agarose bead) to specifically adsorb proteins binding the ligand from solution. After washing off the unbound material, the specifically bound proteins can be competitively eluted by another ligand or eluted by extremes of pH or salt concentration. In principle, affinity chromatography offers a method for achieving extremely large extents of both purification and concentration in a single step. Thus it can overcome the barriers of extremely low concentration and low amount that hampers purification of most receptors. It has the further advantage in that it depends on the ligand-binding properties of the protein rather than on its size, charge, shape, or density as conventional purification techniques do. Affinity chromatography is especially useful for purification of detergent solubilized membrane proteins that may be part of detergent micelles in which the uniformity of the micelles could obscure differences in bulk properties of the proteins to be separated or otherwise hamper conventional techniques.

The methods of affinity chromatography have been extensively reviewed (4). Thus only a few general comments about the method will be presented here. First, it is necessary to find a ligand that has both high affinity and high specificity for binding to the receptor. This ligand must also have a readily reactive functional group (typically an amino group) in a portion of the molecule that is not critical to binding. This functional group is used to attach the ligand to the insoluble support. Frequently a sidearm is required between the ligand and the support in order to provide sufficient space between the support and the ligand to permit the protein to bind. Supports of agarose, acrylamide, or glass beads are used. A desirable support has the properties of ease in conjugation to the sidearm or ligand, of showing little nonspecific binding of proteins, and of mechanical and chemical stability so that it will not slowly "bleed off" ligand or ligand–receptor conjugates. If an affinity adsorbent can be constructed that specifically adsorbs a solubilized receptor from solution, then the next step is to elute the bound receptor. It must be borne in mind that the specificity of affinity chromatography will be limited by the specificities of the attached ligand. For example, affinity columns containing synthetic cholinergic ligands bind both acetylcholine receptors and acetylcholine esterase (54). These two proteins are readily distinguishable after elution, but this may not always be the case. Specific elution by competition with a ligand differing in structure from the ligand conjugated to the support offers a second step of affinity purification. If this cannot be achieved, or is unnecessary, then elution is often achieved using extremes of pH or ionic strength. This is intended to overcome the ligand–protein interactions, but extremes of pH and ionic strength have the potential disadvantage that denaturation of the protein may occur. In some cases the ligand–protein binding may be of such high affinity that only denaturing conditions such as the use of sodium dodecylsulfate will achieve elution. This approach has the huge disadvantage that the functional activity of the eluted protein cannot be determined.

B. Purification of the Acetylcholine Receptor on Toxin–Agarose

The specific case of purification of the acetylcholine receptor by affinity chromatography on an adsorbent of toxin conjugated to agarose will be considered step by step as an illustration. Using this method, in 2 days it is possible to purify receptor from the electric organs of torpedo (at a yield of 60%) and electrophorus (30 to 40% yield) and the muscles of rats and calves (~15% yield) (32,35,37). *Naja naja* toxin 3 (26) has nearly ideal properties for a ligand to be used in affinity chromatography. Unlike synthetic acetylcholine analogues, its high-affinity binding is almost exclusively to the acetylcholine receptor. Purification of this small protein toxin is far easier and less expensive than synthesis of an acetylcholine analog, and it is easily conjugated to cyanogen bromide-activated agarose beads without the need of a spacer arm. The main problem with toxin is that its affinity for receptor is so great that elution may be difficult. Experiments have indicated that the best elution is obtained using conjugates prepared using agarose beads activated by cyanogen bromide using NaOH titration during the reaction (4), by performing the coupling step at pH 9.5 in bicarbonate buffer, and by using less than 0.5 mg/ml (62 nmol/ml) toxin. The resulting conjugates have a binding capacity for receptor of 2 to 4 nmol/ml, indicating that much of the toxin is inactivated or inaccessible to receptor. Epichlorohydrin crosslinked agarose (C14B, Pharmacia) is used to minimize bleeding off of toxin, but binding capacity diminishes significantly after 6 or 7 uses.

Receptor is solubilized in detergent from electric organ or muscle crude membrane preparations at 0 to 4°C. For example, torpedo electric organ tissue and 3 volumes of buffer containing protease inhibitors is homogenized in a Waring blender for 1 min. After centrifugation for 30 min at $10^5 \times g$, the supernate containing soluble components is discarded. The pellet is resuspended in 3 volumes of buffer containing protease inhibitors and then 10% sodium cholate is added to give a final concentration of 1%. After gentle agitation for 1 hr to permit solubilization of receptor, centrifugation is repeated for 30 min at $10^5 \times g$. The supernatant containing solubilized receptor is retained. Extracts of muscle are usually prepared using Triton X-100 instead of cholate, and extraction time may be increased to overnight. For both muscle and electric organ tissue the solutions used for homogenization, extraction, and subsequent handling of receptor usually contain 10 to 20 mM sodium phosphate pH ~7 as buffer, 10 mM sodium azide to inhibit bacterial growth, and 1 mM ethylenediamine tetraacetate, 1 mM phenylmethylsulfonylfluoride to inhibit proteolytic enzymes.

The first step in affinity purification of the acetylcholine receptor on toxin–agarose is to incubate the detergent extract with the toxin–agarose conjugate. This is done batchwise for 1 hr to overnight on a shaker. The high affinity of toxin for receptor permits adequate binding in suspension, unlike the situation occurring when some synthetic ligands are used that must be kept packed in columns to maintain a high local concentration of ligand. Toxin–receptor binding is a rather slow process; thus a long incubation of extract and toxin–agarose is used, especially when receptor is present at low concentration. Batchwise binding has the advantage of preventing the buildup of particulate material that may become trapped if the extract is passed over the adsorbent packed in a column.

The second step of purification is washing the toxin–agarose conjugate, to which receptor is bound, free of extraneous material. This seemingly trivial step is extremely important in that it determines whether or not a homogeneous purified material is obtained. Toxin–agarose can be freed of the particulate fatty material found in extracts from electrophorus electric organ or muscle by collecting the conjugate on a filter and then washing it several times with detergent buffer using a clinical centrifuge for 1 or 2 min to settle the conjugate between washes. The conjugate is then packed into a chromatography column and washed with many volumes of detergent buffer. High salt concentrations and changes of detergent (e.g., from 0.5% Triton to 0.2% sodium cholate) can be used at this point to increase the effectiveness of washing. Washing is complete when no further protein is observed in the eluate.

Elution of receptor from the toxin–agarose is the third step in purification.

Benzoquinonium is a high-affinity receptor antagonist that is useful for competitive elution of receptor. As the benzoquinonium solution (10^{-3} M) elutes from the column of toxin–agarose, it passes through an attached column of DEAE, which binds the eluted receptor because of its net negative charge, but allows the benzoquinonium to pass and be pumped back through the toxin–agarose. Because of the high affinity of binding between receptor and toxin, 3 hr or more at room temperature or overnight at 4° C are allowed for elution.

The fourth step of purification is to wash the unbound benzoquinonium off of the DEAE column, and then to elute the bound receptor with a detergent buffer containing a high salt concentration (0.5 M NaCl). The DEAE column step serves two main functions. It concentrates the receptor slowly eluted from the toxin–agarose, and it separates the eluted receptor from the benzoquinonium used for elution. It could also provide some additional purification.

In the case of acetylcholine receptor from electric organs, the receptor eluted from DEAE is a homogeneous, pure protein. If this were not the case, then sucrose gradient centrifugation or other techniques could be applied at this point for further purification. If such techniques were to be applied before the purification and concentration achieved by affinity chromatography, they would be of little use. This affinity chromatographic method is both easy and fast. The speed helps minimize proteolysis and other forms of denaturation that may accrue during purification.

As a preliminary step before affinity chromatography on toxin–agarose, a concanavallin A-agarose column has been used to partially purify acetylcholine receptor from muscle (12). Concanavallin binds to certain carbohydrate residues on the receptor glycoprotein. Specific elution was achieved using α-methyl mannoside. Lectin affinity columns in addition to ligand affinity columns might prove useful in the purification of many receptors.

Affinity chromatographic purification of other neurotransmitter receptors may not be so easy as purification of the acetylcholine receptor. Ligands as specific as toxin may not be available, and the degree of purification required may be much larger than is required with electric organs. Thus substantial purification by conventional methods may be required subsequent to affinity chromatography.

IV. CHARACTERIZATION

Three basic types of problems must be dealt with in characterizing what is thought to be a purified receptor. First, the homogeneity of the product must be determined, and second, it must be determined whether this homogeneous purified component is part of the physiologically significant receptor. Third, the chemical composition and physical properties of the material must be defined.

Homogeneity is usually tested by determining whether or not the purified material behaves as a single component on sucrose gradient centrifugation, gel filtration chromatography, electrophoresis, or immunoprecipitation. If more than one component can be resolved by any of these techniques, then the technique can be used to further purify the component thought to be the receptor. The application of these types of techniques to the acetylcholine receptor will be briefly reviewed as an example. Centrifugation of affinity-purified acetylcholine receptor reveals a single toxin-binding component sedimenting at approximately 9.5 S in both muscle and electrophorus electric organ extracts (3,19,32); however, torpedo electric organ extracts also contain a component corresponding to a dimer of this size (19,29,54). The dimer is formed by disulfide bonds between the largest of four polypeptide chains composing each monomer (2). Treatment of dimers with reducing agents (2) or with trypsin (29) produces monomers. It is possible that dimers or higher multimers of receptor may be the native form in muscle or electrophorus tissue as well, but that reduction or proteolysis during purification has obscured their presence. Finding a single homogeneous component becomes even more complex when electrophoresis is used to resolve components in affinity-purified acetylcholine receptor preparations. Electrophoresis of receptor from torpedo in the presence of a nondenaturing detergent such as Triton X-100 reveals the same two components that can be resolved by centrifugation on sucrose gradients or gel filtration (19). Electrophoresis in the presence of the denaturing detergent sodium dodecyl sulfate and the reducing agent β-mercaptoethanol reveals that both monomers and dimers are composed of the same four polypeptide chains of apparent mw 64,000, 57,000, 49,500, and 38,000 (19,54). The 38,000 chain can be affinity labeled with the acetylcholine analog MBTA; thus this chain is known to contribute residues to the acetylcholine binding site of the receptor (19). But what about the other three chains? Are they also components of the receptor macromolecule composing the ionophore or other functionally important parts, or are they copurifying contaminants trapped in detergent micelles along with the receptor? This debate is still continuing. Recently it was reported that receptor-rich membrane fragments purified from torpedo electric organ contained high ratios of the 38,000 chain compared to the others, and it was suggested that the other chains were contaminants (63). However, it is also known that receptor is very susceptible to proteolysis. For example, mild trypsinization of electrophorus receptor produces proteolytic fragments all of which have apparent mw of less than 42,000, yet toxin binding capacity of the receptor is not reduced (50). Each of the polypeptide chains composing torpedo receptor have been purified by preparative electrophoresis (35). Rats immunized with any of the four chains developed an autoimmune response that cross-reacted *in vivo* with receptor in rat muscle, causing experimental autoimmune myasthenia gravis (34). The antisera raised to each chain cross-reacted *in vitro* with receptor extracted from human muscle, and the reaction of each antiserum was specifically inhibited by preincubation with the appropriate chain from torpedo receptor. This is strong evidence that components analogous to all four chains of torpedo receptor are conserved through evolution because they are important components of receptor structure. Obviously, establishing homogeneity of a purified receptor is a process that may continue for some years after the initial purification is achieved.

Establishing the identity of a purified component with the physiologically significant receptor is a difficult problem. The receptor must be distinguished not only from completely extraneous contaminants, but also from other proteins with similar binding sites involved, for example, in transmitter synthesis, destruction, or transport that might copurify by affinity chromatography. Since solubilization or purification of these proteins might alter their binding properties, the ligand-binding profile used to distinguish these sites *in situ* may no longer be entirely applicable. The enzymatic, transport, or other effector component associated with each protein that might show some affinity for the transmitter is the critical feature for identifying which component is the physiologically significant receptor molecule. Ideally the purified component should be reconstituted into an artificial membrane and shown to regulate ion conductance, or whatever elemental event is regulated by the receptor *in vivo,* in response to appropriate ligands applied to the artificial membrane. Reconstitution of the receptor for acetylcholine or any other neurotransmitter receptor has not been reproducibly achieved, despite a number of claims (41,47). In addition to problems of methodology for achieving reconstitution, another problem besetting reconstitution is that receptor and effector may not be part of the same macromolecule and may be separated during solubilization. This is clearly true in cases involving the adrenergic receptor and the adenylcyclase that it regulates (46,66). Still another problem is that the effector component of a receptor, such as an ionophore, may be present in a purified component but it may be denatured. Affinity chromatography is directed toward the ligand-binding portion of the receptor, without regard for the presence or functional integrity of any associated effector. The processes of solubilization and purification may also alter the binding properties of the receptor. The ligand-binding properties of the acetylcholine receptor, for example, are sensitive to perturbation by agents such as detergents and local anesthetics and also by the history of ligand binding (3). Affinity chromatography might well leave a receptor in a conformation corresponding to a desensitized receptor *in vivo,* or perhaps not quite corresponding to anything seen *in vivo* (3).

How then can identity be established? Ligand-binding properties of the purified material as compared to those of the receptor are very important (3,54). Affinity labeling is very useful (19). An approach taken in the case of the acetylcholine receptor was to prepare antibodies against the purified component and demonstrate that these antibodies specifically inhibited activity of the receptor in intact electric organ cells (51). In this particular case, immunization with receptor also produced cross reaction with muscle acetylcholine receptors *in vivo* (48), providing further proof of the identity of the component. Whether or not immunization with other purified receptors will produce cross reaction *in vivo* remains to be determined, but is not unlikely. Immunization of rabbits with prolactin receptors did not produce an obvious autoimmune response (59); however, naturally occurring antibodies to acetylcholine receptors are pathogenic factors in myasthenia gravis (31), as are antibodies to thyrotropin receptors in Grave's disease (52), or insulin receptors in certain types of insulin-resistant diabetes (11). Antibodies to membrane components may not inhibit their function (23). In this case, the antibodies labeled with ^{125}I, peroxidase (8), or fluorescine might be used to localize the purified component in tissue in order to determine if this correlates with the location expected for the physiologically significant receptor. In any case, immunohistochemical localization of a receptor is likely to provide valuable information.

Determination of the physical properties of the purified receptor is a two-stage process. First, the elementary physical properties must be determined; for example, is the receptor a protein? What size are its polypeptide components, and what is their stoichiometry in the receptor macromolecule? What is the amino acid, carbohydrate, and lipid composition? Second, once these properties have been delineated, it remains to be determined how these structures function during the regulation of the transducer by ligand binding. For example, what polypeptide chain or chains form the ligand-binding site or the ionophore? Are there areas of these chains responsible for receptor–receptor or receptor–nerve interactions? Does ligand binding induce conformation changes in the molecule? Do these conformational changes regulate the ionophore or cyclase or other effector? How? How does the effector work? Determination of the structural basis for receptor function is clearly a long and difficult project, only barely begun even in the case of the acetylcholine receptor.

Electrophoresis of proteins dissociated in sodium dodecyl sulfate on acrylamide gels in one (24) or two dimensions (45) is a method suited to preliminary characterization of receptors. The amount of sample required, particularly when radiolabeled proteins are used, is small enough to be within the range of that attainable with receptors. Also, the resolution of the technique is extremely good. A two-dimensional gel employing isoelectric focusing in the first dimension and electrophoresis in sodium dodecyl sulfate in the second dimension can, from a single sample of a few micrograms, provide information on purity, number, and apparent molecular weight of polypeptide components, rough stoichiometry, and isoelectric point. By appropriate staining of the gel, the presence of carbohydrate on the polypeptides can be detected. Even the pattern of peptides that can be generated by trypsin-catalyzed hydrolysis of a polypeptide chain can be determined using a single gel slice (7). Other subtle microtechniques are also available for studying micro amounts of protein resolved by electrophoresis on gels.

Determination of the functional roles of the structural components of receptors is more difficult, and largely unprecedented. Ideally, reconstitution of purified receptor into an artificial membrane would be part of such a study. The conditions required for reconstitution would provide information about, for example, lipid cofactor requirements for receptor function. Artificial planar lipid bilayer membranes (44) have the potential advantage that effects of ligands on receptor-mediated ion conductances could be measured electrically for direct comparison with electrophysiological measures made *in vivo.* Artificial lipid monolayer vesicles have the potential advantages of having been used successfully in the reconstitution of several membrane protein systems (14,53) and are convenient for associated biochemical studies. Both approaches to reconstitution have the disadvantage of not having been shown, convincingly and reproducibly, to work for the acetylcholine receptor, despite many claims. This does not mean that functional studies of purified receptor are limited to the binding properties of the protein in detergent micelles. Because the acetylcholine receptor is densely packed in the tips of folds in the postsynaptic membrane, membrane vesicles containing at least one-half of their protein as acetylcholine receptor can be purified (3,54). Receptor function is retained in these vesicles and can be measured as carbamylcholine-sensitive flux of $^{22}Na^{+}$ across the vesicle membrane (3). Another approach to relating structure of purified receptor to functional properties of the receptor in intact cells is immunologic. It is known that antibodies to purified acetylcholine receptor affect receptor-mediated conductance changes in intact cells (15,51). Antibodies also affect receptor metabolism (15). By preparing antibodies to single parts of the purified receptor molecule and testing their effect on receptor function in intact cells it may be possible to determine the functional role of each part. By determining which parts of polypeptide chains are accessible to antibody binding in the cell, orientation of polypeptide chains in the membrane can be determined. Some progress has been made on this type of study (35). It might be possible using antibodies as probes to disturb receptor function, such as neurotrophic interactions, which could not be adequately modeled in artificial lipid bilayers. Also, because there is interspecies cross reaction of acetylcholine receptors (33,37,49), antibodies made to receptor from a readily accessible source such as electric organ can be used to study receptors from a much less tractable source such as muscle (35). Similar methods should be applicable to the study of receptors for other neurotransmitters.

V. STUDIES WITH ANTIBODIES

A. Naturally Occurring Antireceptor Antibodies

The antibodies to skeletal muscle acetylcholine receptors found in the sera of patients with myasthenia gravis (30) are not the only naturally occurring antibodies to receptors known. Certain patients with insulin-resistant diabetes contain antibodies to insulin receptors (11). Antibodies to thyrotropin-stimulating hormone receptors are pathogenic agents in Grave's disease (52,62). No doubt a number of other receptors are the objects of autoimmune diseases. Study of these antibodies should result in providing at least as much information about these various receptors as it does about the pathologies of the various diseases involved.

Antibodies to receptors of several types may be involved in autoimmune diseases as yet unrecognized. If antibodies to a receptor were suspected as pathogenic agents in a disease of unknown cause, then it might be possible to detect these antibodies in the sera of patients by testing for the ability of these sera to inhibit ligand binding to cells (11) or a crude extract of receptor (52,62), or by immunoprecipitation of receptor–ligand complexes (30). Naturally occurring antireceptor antibodies could prove very useful reagents for identifying a receptor during its purification and for characterization of the purified molecule.

B. Experimental Autoimmune Myasthenia Gravis

Experimental autoimmune myasthenia gravis (EAMG) is a model of human MG produced by immunizing animals with acetylcholine receptor purified from electric organs (28) or even genetically identical muscle (33). Rats given a single injection of receptor (1 to 100 μg) in complete Freund's adjuvant undergo two phases of EAMG: first a transient acute phase, and then a chronic phase.

During the acute phase of EAMG, 8 to 11 days after immunization, muscular weakness occurs owing to impairment of neuromuscular transmission by a phagocytic invasion of the endplate (10). At this time concentration of antibodies in serum recognizing muscle receptor is low (34). The initial event in the acute phase is binding of antibodies to receptors in the postsynaptic membrane, which allows fixation of complement that causes focal destruction of the tips of the postjunctional folds where receptor is most concentrated. Probably breakdown products of complement act as trophic factors inducing the migration of macrophages to the endplate. The phagocytes ingest the postsynaptic membrane, resulting in functional denervation (25). For unknown reasons, the phagocytic invasion is transient. There is a net loss of receptor during the acute phase followed by an overshoot in receptor content owing to repair synthesis and denervation hypersensitivity (34).

By the time chronic weakness appears, 28 to 30 days after immunization, receptor content has decreased to one-third or so of normal, and more than one-half of the receptors that remain have antibodies bound. In chronic EAMG, postsynaptic membrane structure is greatly simplified and no phagocytes are seen (10). Receptor can be localized electronmicroscopically with toxin–peroxidase conjugates (9), bound antibody with protein A–peroxidase conjugates (8), and the C3 component of complement with anti-C3–peroxidase conjugates (8). Miniature endplate potentials of small amptitude (25) and decrementing electromyograms are observed (58). Receptor loss in these animals is probably mediated both by complement dependent focal destruction of the postsynaptic membrane and by antigenic modulation of the acetylcholine receptor (15). It can be demonstrated that antibodies to receptor increase the rate of receptor destruction in cultured muscle cells (15). Antibodies to receptor from a rat with chronic EAMG can passively transfer an acute form of EAMG to a normal rat (36). Antibodies to receptor added to muscle (15) or electric organ cells (51) under conditions where neither complement, phagocytes, nor modulation occur, directly inhibit receptor activity, but only partially.

C. Production, Assay, and Use of Antibodies to the Acetylcholine Receptor

Two extremely good reasons for the use of antibodies in the study of receptors are (a) that antibodies to a receptor protein can be obtained in relatively large amounts by immunization with even microgram quantities of receptor, and (b) that antibodies may provide the only available probes for parts of the receptor macromolecule outside the ligand binding site. In the case of the acetylcholine receptor, virtually none of the antibodies raised against it are directed at the acetylcholine binding site (29).

Antisera to acetylcholine receptors have been raised like antibodies to other purified proteins. Purified receptor, in as little detergent as possible, is emulsified with complete Freund's adjuvant and injected intradermally at multiple sites (28). Pertussis vaccine may be used as an additional adjuvant (28). Many species have been immunized with purified receptor including rabbits (48), rats (34), mice (13), guinea pigs (28), goats (33), and monkeys (65). The amount of receptor injected and the injection schedule have varied widely according to the tastes of the investigators and the practical demands presented by differences in the development of EAMG depending on the dose of receptor or the species immunized. Rats given a single injection containing 1 μg of torpedo receptor and even less rat muscle receptor develop EAMG, but higher doses (10 to 100 μg) and booster immunizations at approximately 2-week intervals are more effective at producing high antibody titers.

Radioimmune assay of antibodies to the acetylcholine receptor is simple (30,51). ^{125}I toxin labeled receptor can be used as antigen. Purification of the antigen is unnecessary because the specificity resides in the specificity of toxin–receptor binding. Normal serum and inhibition of ^{125}I-toxin binding by receptor ligands provide specificity controls. Tubes containing a fixed amount of toxin-labeled receptor are incubated overnight with increasing amounts of a serum dilution. In the morning, complexes of ^{125} I-toxin–receptor–antibody together with carrier antibody are precipitated with anti-antibody, and the radioactivity in the washed pellets is determined. The result is a curve in which the amount of ^{125}I–toxin–receptor precipitated is initially directly proportional to the amount of antiserum added. The curve plateaus when all the ^{125}I-toxin–receptor present has been precipitated. Antibody titer measured in moles of ^{125}I-toxin-binding sites precipitated per liter of serum is obtained from the initial slope of the curve. Receptor concentration measured in moles ^{125}I-toxin-binding sites per liter is obtained from the plateau value of the curve. Receptor polypeptide chains can be assayed by inhibition of antibody binding to ^{125}I-toxin-labeled receptor (35).

Antibodies to receptor are highly species specific (32,36). Usually only 1 to 2% of the antibodies to torpedo receptor in the serum of a rat will also recognize receptor from rat muscle. But, as has been described, the absolute amount of these antibodies in a rat's serum (typically 50 to 200 $\times 10^{-11}$ mol/rat with severe chronic EAMG) compared with the small amount of receptor in a normal rat (5×10^{-11} mol/rat) is sufficient to wreak havoc on neuromuscular transmission. The species specificity of these antibodies could, in principle, be used to compare receptors from related species (33).

In summary, antibodies to acetylcholine receptors have been used in a number of ways, including: (a) to assay receptor concentration (34), (b) to inhibit receptor activity (51), (c) to effect a disease model (36,48), (d) to increase receptor degradation (15), (e) to compare the structure of receptors from various sources (33), (f) to localize receptor (8), (g) to prove that isolated receptor is part of the physiologically significant receptor (51), and (h) to prove that the polypeptide chains in purified receptor are each part of the physiologically significant receptor (35). This list is growing constantly, and testifies to the usefulness of antibodies as probes for receptor studies both *in vitro* and *in vivo.*

In the future it is probable that antireceptor antibodies will be used in still other ways in receptor studies. For example, antibodies to defined regions of the receptor molecule could be used to test the role of these regions in receptor function *in vivo.* Or antibodies to receptor along with complement might be used to select receptor-minus mutants in cell lines. Rigorous biochemical study of neurotransmitter receptors is difficult; thus it is likely that as useful a tool as antibodies will find a use in the study of many receptors.

VI. SUMMARY

Purification of neurotransmitter receptors is just beginning. The acetylcholine receptor protein is the only case in which purification has been achieved and characterization begun, so it naturally provides a model for future studies with other receptors. Certain barriers to biochemical studies are common to most neurotransmitter receptors. These include low amounts of receptor in tissue, solubilization of the receptor from the membrane in a native conformation, achieving large factors of concentration and purification while retaining high yield, and testing the homogeneity and physiological significance of the purified component. In this chapter the approaches taken to these problems in the case of the acetylcholine receptor have been reviewed, with comments on other approaches that might be used. The use of mild detergents to solubilize receptors and of affinity chromatography for purification are considered likely to be used in the study of most receptors, but the critical nuances of method are likely to vary widely with the demands of each system. The importance of dealing with receptors as complex macromolecules with other functions in addition to ligand binding is emphasized, particularly in reference to preserving them from degradation and denaturation during purification. Finally the value of using antireceptor antibodies in studies of receptor structure and function has been stressed.

ACKNOWLEDGMENT

Research in the author's laboratory has been supported by the National Institutes of Health (NS11323) and by the Muscular Dystrophy Association.

VII. REFERENCES

1. Berg, D. K., Kelley, R. B., Sargent, P. B., Williamson, P., and Hall, Z. W. (1972): Binding of α-bungarotoxin to acetylcholine receptors in mammalian muscle. *Proc. Natl. Acad. Sci. USA,* 69:147–151.
2. Chang, H. W., and Bock, E. (1977): Molecular forms of the acetylcholine receptor: Effects of calcium ions and a sulfhydryl reagent on the occurrence of oligomers. *Biochemistry,* 16:4513–4520.
3. Changeux, J. P., Benedetti, L., Bourgeois, J. P., Brisson, A., Cartaud, J., Devaus, P., Grunhangen, H., Moreau, M., Popot, J., Sobel, A., and Weber, M. (1976): Some structural properties of the cholinergic receptor protein in its membrane environment relevant to its function as a pharmacological receptor. *Cold Spring Harbor Symp. Quant. Biol.,* 40:211–230.
4. Cuatrecasas, P., and Anfinsen, C. B. (1971): Affinity chromatography. *Annu. Rev. Biochem.,* 40:259–278.
5. Das, M., Miyakawa, T., Fox, C. F., Pruss, R. M., Aharonov, A., and Herschman, H. R. (1977): Specific radiolabeling of a cell surface receptor for epidermal growth factor. *Proc. Natl. Acad. Sci. USA,* 74:2790–2794.
6. Devreotes, P. N., and Fambrough, D. M. (1975): Acetylcholine receptor turnover in membranes of developing muscle fibers. *J. Cell. Biol.,* 65:335–358.
7. Elder, J. H., Pickett, R. A., Hampton, J., and Lerner, R. A. (1977): Radioiodination of proteins in single acrylamide gel slices. *J. Biol. Chem.,* 252:6510–6515.
8. Engel, A., Lambert, E., and Howard, G. (1977): Localization of acetylcholine receptors, antibodies, and complement at endplates of patients with myasthenia gravis. *Mayo Clin. Proc.,* 52:267–280.
9. Engel, A. G., Lindstrom, J. M., Lambert, E. H., and Lennon, V. A. (1977): Ultra-structural localization of the acetylcholine receptor in myasthenia gravis and its experimental autoimmune model. *Neurology (Minneap),* 27:307–315.
10. Engel, A., Tsujihata, M., Lindstrom, J., and Lennon, V. (1976): End-plate fine structure in myasthenia gravis and in experimental autoimmune myasthenia gravis. *Ann. NY Acad. Sci.,* 274:60–79.
11. Flier, J., Kahn, C. R., Jarrett, D. B., and Roth, J. (1976): The immunology of the insulin receptor. *Immunol. Commun.,* 5:361–373.
12. Froehner, S., Karlin, A., and Hall, Z. (1977): Affinity alkylation labels two subunits of reduced acetylcholine receptor from mammalian muscle. *Proc. Natl. Acad. Sci. USA,* 74:4685–4688.
13. Fuchs, S., Nevo, D., and Tarrab-Hazdai, R. (1976): Strain differences in the autoimmune response of mice to acetylcholine receptors. *Nature (Lond),* 263:329–330.
14. Goldin, S. M. (1977): Active transport of sodium and potassium ions by the sodium and potassium ion-activated adenosine triphosphatase from renal medulla. *J. Biol. Chem.,* 252:5630–5642.
15. Heinemann, S., Bevan, S., Kullberg, R., Lindstrom, J., and Rice, J. (1977): Modulation of the acetylcholine receptor by anti-receptor antibody. *Proc. Natl. Acad. Sci. USA,* 74:3090–3094.
16. Helenius, A., and Simons, K. (1975): Solubilization of membranes by detergents. *Biochim. Biophys. Acta,* 415:29–79.
17. Karlin, A., and Cowburn, D. (1973): The affinity-labeling of partially purified acetylcholine receptor from electric tissue of Electrophorus. *Proc. Natl. Acad. Sci. USA,* 70:3636–3640.
18. Karlin, A., Prives, J., Deal, W., and Winnik, M. (1971): Affinity labeling of the acetylcholine receptor in electroplax. *J. Mol. Biol.,* 61:175–188.
19. Karlin, A., Weill, C. L., McNamee, M. G., and Valderrama, R. (1976): Facets of the structures of acetylcholine receptors from Electrophorus and Torpedo. *Cold Spring Harbor Symp. Quant. Biol.,* 40:203–210.

20. Kasai, M., and Changeux, J. P. (1971): In vitro excitation of purified membrane fragments by cholinergic agonists. I. Pharmacological properties of the excitable membrane fragments. *J. Membr. Biol.,* 6:1–23.
21. Katz, B., and Miledi, R. (1972): The statistical nature of the acetylcholine potential and its molecular components. *J. Physiol. (Lond),* 224:665–699.
22. Kyte, J. (1971): Purification of the sodium- and potassium-dependent adenosine triphosphatase from canine renal medulla. *J. Biol. Chem.,* 246:4157–4165.
23. Kyte, J. (1974): The reactions of ($Na^+ + K^+$) adenosine triphosphatase with specific antibodies: Implications for the mechanism of active transport. *J. Biol. Chem.,* 249:3652–3660.
24. Laemmli, U. (1970): Cleavage of structural proteins during the assembly of the head of bacteriophage T4. *Nature (Lond),* 227:680–685.
25. Lambert, E., Lindstrom, J., and Lennon, V. (1976): Endplate potentials in experimental autoimmune myasthenia. *Ann. NY Acad. Sci.,* 274:300–318.
26. Lee, C. Y. (1972): Chemistry and pharmacology of polypeptide toxins in snake venoms. *Annu. Rev. Pharmacol.,* 12:265–286.
27. Lee, C. Y., Tseng, L. F., and Chiu, T. H. (1967): Influence of denervation on localization of neurotoxins from clapid venoms in rat diaphragms. *Nature (Lond),* 215:1177–1178.
28. Lennon, V. A., Lindstrom, J. M., and Seybold, M. E. (1975): Experimental autoimmune myasthenia: A model of myasthenia gravis in rats and guinea pigs. *J. Exp. Med.,* 141:1365–1375.
29. Lindstrom, J. (1976): Immunological studies of acetylcholine receptors. *J. Supramol. Struct.,* 4:389–403.
30. Lindstrom, J. (1977): An assay for antibodies to human acetylcholine receptor in serum from patients with myasthenia gravis. *J. Clin. Immunol. Immunopathol.,* 7:36–43.
31. Lindstrom, J. (1977): Pathological mechanisms in myasthenia gravis and its animal model, experimental autoimmune myasthenia gravis. In: *The Biochemistry of Myasthenia Gravis and Muscular Dystrophy,* edited by R. Marchbanks and G. Lunt, pp. 135–156. Academic Press, New York.
32. Lindstrom, J., and Patrick, J. (1974): Purification of the acetylcholine receptor by affinity chromatography. In: *Synaptic Transmission and Neuronal Interaction,* edited by M. V. L. Bennett, pp. 191–216. Raven Press, New York.
33. Lindstrom, J., Campbell, M., and Nave, B. (1977): Specificities of antibodies to acetylcholine receptors. *Muscle and Nerve,* 1:140–145.
34. Lindstrom, J. M., Einarson, B., Lennon, V. A., and Seybold, M. E. (1976): Pathological mechanisms in EAMG I: Immunogenicity of syngeneic muscle acetylcholine receptor and quantitative extraction of receptor and antibody-receptor complexes from muscles of rats with experimental autoimmune myasthenia gravis. *J. Exp. Med.,* 144:726–738.
35. Lindstrom, J., Einarson, B., and Merlie, J. (1977): Immunization of rats with polypeptide chains from Torpedo acetylcholine receptor causes an autoimmune response to receptors in rat muscle. *Proc. Natl. Acad. Sci. USA,* 75:769–773.
36. Lindstrom, J. M., Engel, A. G., Seybold, M. E., Lennon, V. A., and Lambert, E. H. (1976): Pathological mechanisms in EAMG II: Passive transfer of experimental autoimmune myasthenia gravis in rats with anti-acetylcholine receptor antibodies. *J. Exp. Med.,* 144:739–753.
37. Lindstrom, J., Lennon, V., Seybold, M., and Whittingham, S. (1976): Experimental autoimmune myasthenia gravis and myasthenia gravis: Biochemical and immunochemical aspects. *Ann. NY Acad. Sci.,* 274:254–274.
38. Lwebuga-Mukasa, J. S., Lappi, S., and Taylor, P. (1976): Molecular forms of acetylcholinesterase from Torpedo californica: Their relationship to synaptic membranes. *Biochemistry,* 15:1425–1434.
39. Marchesi, V. T. (1975): The structure and orientation of a membrane protein. In: *Cell Membranes,* edited by G. Weissmann and R. Claiborne. H. P. Publishing Co., New York.
40. Marchesi, V. T., and Andrews, E. P. (1971): Glycoproteins isolated from cell membranes with lithium diiodosalicylate. *Science,* 174:1247–1248.
41. Michaelson, D., and Raftery, M. A. (1974): Purified acetylcholine receptor: Its reconstitution to a chemically excitable membrane. *Proc. Natl. Acad. Sci. USA,* 71:4768–4772.
42. Miledi, R., Molinoff, P., and Potter, L. T. (1971): Isolation of the cholinergic receptor protein of Torpedo electric tissue. *Nature (Lond),* 229:554–557.
43. Monsour, N., Eldefrawi, M., and Eldefrawi, A. (1977): Isolation of putative acetylcholine receptor proteins from housefly brain. *Biochemistry,* 16:4126–4132.

44. Montal, M. (1974): Formation of bimolecular membranes from lipid monolayers. *Methods Enzymol.,* 32:545–556.
45. O'Farrell, P. H. (1975): High resolution two-dimensional electrophoresis of proteins. *J. Biol. Chem.,* 250:4007–4021.
46. Orly, J., and Schramm, J. (1976): Coupling of catecholamine receptor from one cell with adenylate cyclase from another cell by fusion. *Proc. Natl. Acad. Sci. USA,* 73:4410–4414.
47. Parisi, M., Reader, T. A., and De Robertis, E. (1972): Conductance properties of artificial lipidic membranes containing a proteolipid from Electrophorus. *J. Gen. Physiol.,* 60:454–470.
48. Patrick, J., and Lindstrom, J. (1973): Autoimmune response to acetylcholine receptor. *Science,* 180:871–872.
49. Patrick, J., and Stallcup, B. (1977): α-Bungarotoxin binding and cholinergic receptor function on a rat sympatheic nerve line. *J. Biol. Chem.,* 74:4689–4692.
50. Patrick, J., Boulter, J., and O'Brien, J. (1975): An acetylcholine receptor preparation lacking the 42,000 dalton component. *Biochem. Biophys. Res. Commun.,* 64:219–225.
51. Patrick, J., Lindstrom, J., Culp, B., and McMillan, J. (1973): Studies on purified eel acetylcholine receptor and anti-acetylcholine receptor antibody. *Proc. Natl. Acad. Sci. USA,* 70:3334–3338.
52. Peterson, V. B., Dawes, P. J. D., Smith, B. R., and Hall, R. (1977): The interaction of thyroid-stimulating antibodies with solubilized human thyrotropin receptors. *FEBS Lett.,* 93:63–67.
53. Racker, E. (1975): Reconstitution of membranes. In: *Proceedings of the Tenth FEBS Meeting,* pp. 25–34.
54. Raftery, M. A., Vandlen, R. L., Reed, K. L., and Lee, R. (1976): Characterization of Torpedo californica acetylcholine receptor: Its subunit composition and ligand binding properties. *Cold Spring Harbor Symp. Quant. Biol.,* 40:193–202.
55. Rieger, F., Bon, S., Massoulie, J., Cartaud, J., Picard, B., and Benda, P. (1972): Torpedo marmorata acetylcholinesterase; a comparison with the Electrophorus electricus enzyme. *Eur. J. Biochem.,* 58:513–521.
56. Ruoho, A., Kiefer, H., Ryder, P., and Singer, S. J., (1973): The mechanism of photoaffinity labeling. *Proc. Natl. Acad. Sci. USA,* 70:2567–2571.
57. Schmidt, J., and Raftery, M. (1973): A simple assay for the study of solubilized acetylcholine receptors. *Anal. Biochem.,* 52:349–354.
58. Seybold, M., Lambert, E., Lennon, V., and Lindstrom, J. (1976): Experimental autoimmune myasthenia gravis: Clinical, neurophysiologic, and pharmacologic aspects. *Ann. NY Acad. Sci.,* 274:275–282.
59. Shiu, R. P. C., and Friesen, H. G. (1976): Blockade of prolactin action by an antiserum to its receptors. *Science,* 192:259–261.
60. Singer, S. J. (1967): Covalent labeling of active sites. *Adv. Protein Chem.,* 22:1–53.
61. Singer, S. J., and Nicolson, G. L. (1972): The fluid mosaic model of the structure of cell membranes. *Science,* 175:720–731.
62. Smith, B. R. (1976): Immunology of the thyrotropin receptor. *Immunol. Commun.,* 5:345–260.
63. Sobel, A., Weber, M., and Changeux, J. P. (1977): Large-scale purification of the acetylcholine-receptor protein in its membrane-bound and detergent-extracted forms from Torpedo marmorata electric organ. *Eur. J. Biochem.,* 80:215–224.
64. Tanford, C., and Reynolds, J. (1976): Characterization of membrane proteins in detergent solutions. *Biochim. Biophys. Acta,* 457:133–170.
65. Tarrab-Hazdai, R., Aharonov, A., Silman, I., Fuchs, S., and Abramsky, O. (1975): Experimental autoimmune myasthenia induced in monkeys by purified acetylcholine receptor. *Nature (Lond),* 256:128–130.
66. Vauquelin, G., Geynet, P., Hanoune, J., and Strosberg, A. (1977): Isolation of adenylate cylcase-free, β adrenergic receptor from turkey erythrocyte membranes by affinity chromatography. *Proc. Natl. Acad. Sci. USA,* 74:3710–3714.
67. Wilson, D. F., Miyata, Y., Erecinska, M., and Vanderkooi, J. M. (1975): An aryl azide suitable for photoaffinity labeling of amino groups in proteins. *Arch. Biochem. Biophys.,* 171:104–107.

Neurotransmitter Receptor Binding, edited by
H. I. Yamamura et al.
Raven Press, New York © 1978.

6

Histochemical Localization of Neurotransmitter Receptors

Michael J. Kuhar

Departments of Pharmacology and Experimental Therapeutics, and Psychiatry and the Behavioral Sciences, The Johns Hopkins University School of Medicine, Baltimore, Maryland 21205

I. INTRODUCTION

A basic question to be asked concerning receptors is, "Where are they localized?" An obvious, direct approach to answering this question is to perform receptor-binding assays with various tissues and tissue subdivisions. However, a problem with this method is that to obtain anatomical information with greater and greater precision and resolution, it is necessary to use smaller and smaller pieces of tissue. Therefore one encounters practical difficulties dealing with dissection time and technique and with obtaining enough tissue for assay. In addition, the *in vitro* binding assays usually involve homogenization of tissue, which destroys anatomical integrity and yields no information about the receptor at the ultrastructural level. These difficulties and deficiencies can be overcome, with varying degrees of success, by using histochemical and cytochemical methods, that is, methods for localizing biochemical elements in morphologically intact tissue sections with the light and the electron microscope.

An advantage of the histochemical approach is that one can sometimes "explain" drug action by identifying the anatomical location of the receptors. For example, opiate receptors are localized to anatomical areas associated with physiologic functions known to be affected by opiate administration (1–3,34). In addition to providing insights about receptor function at a behavioral and physiologic level, these approaches also allow one to define systems with greater precision at the cellular level. Thus it is possible to plan experiments aimed at the metabolism of receptor molecules themselves and at their cellular and biochemical functions. For example, the histochemical localization of cyclic nucleotides permits the demonstration of intraneuronal accumulation of cyclic AMP following catecholamine receptor stimulation (6,24). This information is very important in the construction of our present model of the catecholamine receptor and its association with adenylate cyclase.

Thus these histochemical methods are very powerful, although the techniques are often complex. The purpose of this chapter is to summarize and discuss critical issues in the histochemistry of receptors and to illustrate these issues with some examples. Because of these limited objectives and restrictions in space, an extensive literature review was not attempted.

II. PRELIMINARY CONSIDERATIONS AND METHODS

A problem in describing the histochemical localization of receptors is that the techniques and issues can be quite different depending on the experimental situation. For example, there are a number of important technical differences between light microscopic localization of opiate receptors after intravenous administration of radiolabeled opiates and electron microscopic localization of cholinergic nicotinic receptors on muscle cells in tissue culture with iodinated α-bungarotoxin. On the other hand, there are certain basic issues common to all of these situations and this section will be a discussion of the general problems involved in histochemistry of receptors.

A. Critical Issues in Receptor Labeling for Histochemistry

The methods in receptor histochemistry are indirect; that is, the object localized is a ligand rather than the receptor itself. Therefore one must *selectively* label the receptor, or at least be able to decide which portion of the binding is selective. The critical issues involved in selective binding to neurotransmitter receptors are extensively discussed in Chapters 3 and 4 of this volume. The problems here are similar except that in addition to the requirement of selective binding, the tissue can be processed only in ways that preserve the anatomical structure.

The issue of selectivity is an important one. For example, in localizing receptors by autoradiographic methods with a radioactive ligand, one must be sure that the bulk of the autoradiographic grains observed is in fact associated with receptors rather than with nonspecific tissue sites. Since intact rather than homogenized tissue is utilized for histochemistry, one must be quite careful that the conditions used to obtain a high level of selective binding are the same as the conditions useful for histochemistry. An additional problem is that some other complicating process such as uptake or metabolism of ligand might be occurring. Thus it is worth repeating that one must be certain, with the ligand chosen and under the given experimental conditions, to get a high degree of selective labeling of receptor. In general, extensive *in vitro* biochemical studies with the ligand and tissue of interest are desirable before beginning microscopic studies. This aids the investigator in understanding the particular variables important for a given situation.

How does one approach the problem of obtaining a high degree of selective labeling? The utilization of a ligand with a very high affinity and a correspondingly slow dissociation rate from the receptor is intuitively useful. Table 1 lists some ligands that have been utilized in histochemical studies. There are several means by which selective association of ligand with receptor can be determined. One obvious factor is tissue or region specificity. For example, if *in vitro* biochemical assay shows that a particular brain region has very few receptors compared to another brain region, then after intravenous administration (if this method is chosen for labeling), a similar distribution of ligand should be observed before beginning histochemistry. Also, there should be pharmacologic specificity. For example, in the case of the opiate receptor, one would show that the accumulation of ligand or binding is stereospecific (34). Within the regions of interest, the accumulation of ligand should also be saturable (i.e., specific binding should plateau in spite of increasing doses of ligand), since only a finite number of receptors exist. It is important to check for metabolic degradation by extracting radioactivity from tissue and examining its composition by chromatography. Finally, where possible, it would be highly useful to show some correlation between receptor binding and some function associated with such binding. In later sections, these criteria will be illustrated with some examples.

Assuming that a high degree of selective labeling of receptors within the tissue is attained, the selective association of ligand and receptor must be maintained throughout the procedures utilized for histochemistry. In some cases this may not be a problem. For example, if the ligand is covalently bound, then diffusion of ligand from receptor will not occur. However, some particular step in the histologic process could disrupt this bond or possibly solubilize the entire ligand–receptor complex. Thus with a radioactive ligand one should

TABLE 1. *Some ligands used in receptor histochemistry and their binding characteristics*

Ligand	Receptor	Affinity (K_D-molar)	Reference
α-Naja naja toxin	Cholinergic nicotinic	2×10^{-10}	7,8,41
α-Bungarotoxin	Cholinergic nicotinic	Irreversible	4,16,17,19
Propylbenzilylcholine mustard	Cholinergic muscarinic	Irreversible	9,37
Quinuclidinyl benzilate	Cholinergic muscarinic	10^{-10}	26,27,43,44
Diprenorphine	Opiate, opioid peptide	10^{-10}	1–3,34
Etorphine	Opiate, opioid peptide	10^{-10}	1–3,39,40
9-Aminoacridinpropranolol	β-Adrenergic	3×10^{-8}	31
Spiroperidol	Dopaminergic	3×10^{-10}	13,20,23,28,29

utilize scintillation counting at every step of the histologic process in a series of preliminary experiments to be sure that there is no significant deterioration of binding for any number of reasons. If the ligand is reversibly bound, then diffusion of ligand from receptor is a serious concern. This would be especially important in electron microscopic studies in which even small amounts of diffusion could be important.

B. Visualization of Receptors

There are a number of possible methods for visualizing the ligand in the tissues. Until the present time, the most popular has been autoradiography. A great deal of work has been done with the technique, and because of this background and available expertise, it was relatively easy to adapt these methods to localizing neurotransmitter receptors. A detailed discussion of autoradiographic techniques is beyond the scope of this chapter, but several comprehensive textbooks are available that deal with all aspects of autoradiography (35,36). Briefly, autoradiography is the localization of radioactive molecules in tissues by placing treated tissues in contact with photographic emulsion.

Immunohistochemistry would be useful where antibodies are available to receptors. Immunohistochemical methods have been explored and are described in detail in a number of review articles and texts (12,21).

There are still other possible methods for visualization. For example, a study has appeared utilizing a fluorescent analog of propranolol to localize the β-adrenergic receptor in the rat cerebellum (31). Fluorescence microscopy directly detected the location of the ligand. Other possibilities include utilizing ligands attached to electron-dense molecules, such as ferritin, which can be viewed in the electron microscope.

All of the above methods have important, appropriate controls. For example, autoradiographic experiments must include tests for positive and negative chemography (i.e., tests for artifactual production of or loss of grains), and immunologic experiments include blocked serum (serum with antigen preadsorbed) controls among others. These methodologic controls should be supplemented by specificity controls whenever possible. For example, in experiments visualizing acetylcholine receptors, tissues treated with receptor blockers should be examined to reveal nonspecific localization of ligands and to satisfy the investigator that he does not attach unwarranted significance to binding that may be nonspecific.

The method selected must be adequate to meet the needs and desires of the investigator. Light microscopy has limited resolution and one can only localize receptors to certain regions without getting any reliable information about specific membrane localization. To find out which part of the postsynaptic membrane has a given receptor, one must choose an electron microscopic method because only the electron microscope provides a sufficient level of resolution to obtain this information. However, even electron microscopy has its limits. For example, electron microscopic autoradiography under very optimal conditions has a resolution limited to approximately 1,500 Å (35).

III. SOME EXAMPLES

A. Cholinergic Muscarinic Receptors

1. In Vitro Biochemical Binding Studies

A number of cholinergic muscarinic antagonists have been used as ligands to label this receptor *in vitro.* These include the reversibly binding ligands, 3-quinuclidinyl benzilate (QNB) (43,44), atropine (18), dexetimide (5) and the irreversibly binding antagonist propylbenzilylcholine mustard (PBC) (9). The evidence for the specific receptor labeling by these ligands can be summarized very briefly. When performing binding studies in brain regions or other tissues such as the gastrointestinal tract where it is known that there are cholinergic muscarinic receptors, a high degree of binding that is saturable and that is blocked only by other muscarinic-type drugs and not by a wide variety of other compounds is found. Two of these ligands, quinuclidinyl benzilate and propylbenzilylcholine mustard, have been used in autoradiographic studies to localize cholinergic muscarinic receptors in intact tissue sections with the light microscope.

2. Histochemistry with [^{3}H]3-quinuclidinyl benzilate

The conditions for specific [^{3}H]QNB binding to cholinergic muscarinic receptors *in vitro* are well defined (43). It is also possible to demonstrate specific [^{3}H]QNB binding to muscarinic receptors in rat brain *in vivo* soon after intravenous administration (44). The fact that the accumulation of [^{3}H]QNB in brain after intravenous administration saturates with increasing doses of [^{3}H]QNB, that the regional variation in tissue radioactivity parallels the regional distribution in specific [^{3}H]QNB binding observed by *in vitro* assay, and that 60 to 75% of the accumulated radioactivity can be blocked by pretreatment with atropine, a classic muscarinic antagonist, but not by other noncholinergic compounds, is strong evidence of a selective localization of ligand to receptor. Approximately 85% of total radioactivity in the brain is found in the particulate fraction after homogenization and centrifugation. Because of the high degree of specific [^{3}H]QNB binding *in vivo* it has been possible to perform light microscopic autoradiography to show the distribution of these drug receptor sites (26,27).

Once it is demonstrated that intravenous injection of [^{3}H]QNB results in a specific labeling of receptors, how are these sites "visualized"? Since the ligand is radiolabeled, autoradiography is the logical method of choice. Thus a main experimental problem is how to make tissue sections and appose them to photographic emulsion to reveal the sites of radioactivity. Of course, it is quite important that whatever method is utilized, the bound ligand must not have an opportunity for diffusion. Should significant diffusion occur, the radioactivity will no longer clearly mark the receptor sites. It is fortunate that the diffusion problem has been the subject of much study (36,42), and procedures exist for the autoradiographic localization of diffusible ligands in fresh, frozen unfixed tissue. In these procedures, one has to sacrifice the animal, remove the brain, freeze it onto a microtome chuck, take thin sections (e.g., 4 μm), mount these sections onto emulsion-coated microscope slides, and permit an adequate time to pass for development. The time chosen in the QNB study was approximately 1 month after which time the emulsion was developed, the tissue fixed, stained, and examined in the light microscope.

In these experiments, the autoradiographic grains, which mark the location of [^{3}H]QNB, which under these conditions mark the cholinergic muscarinic receptors, are concentrated in various places in the brain. In Fig. 1A, the arrow marks the dividing line between the corpus callosum and the nucleus caudate–putamen. It is clear that the autoradiographic grains are highly localized to

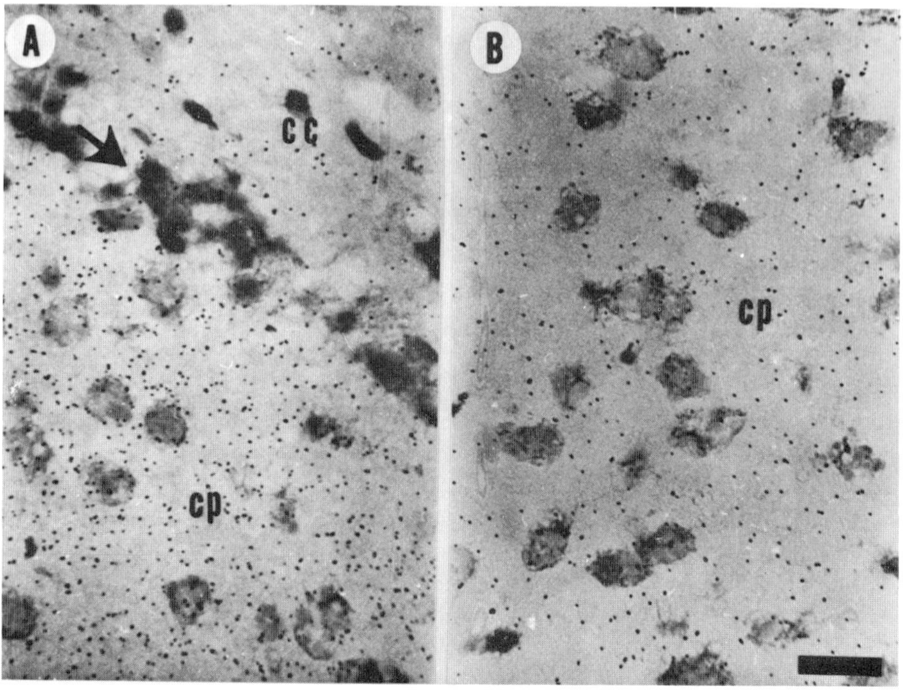

FIG. 1. Light microscopic autoradiographic localization of [^{3}H]quinuclidinyl benzilate (cholinergic muscarinic receptor ligand) in the caudate–putamen (cp) and corpus callosum (CC) of the rat. **A:** An arrow points along the cp–CC border. Note the high grain density in cp rather than CC, a fiber tract. **B:** Tissue from a similarly prepared rat except that it was pretreated with nonradioactive atropine to block specific receptor labeling. Note the significant reduction in grain density in **B** compared to cp in **A.** Bar = 25 μm.

the nucleus caudate–putamen, whereas there is only a background level of grains in the white matter tract, the corpus callosum. It is also important that pretreatment of the animal with atropine, another cholinergic muscarinic drug, prevents the binding of [^{3}H]QNB in this region (Fig. 1B). Under these conditions, the grain density in the nucleus caudate–putamen is about the same as the tissue background density observed in the corpus callosum.

In examining other areas of the brain, autoradiographic grains were observed in association with brain regions known to be rich in cholinergic nerve terminals; these include the hippocampus, cerebral cortex, and nucleus accumbens. Even within these regions, the distribution of autoradiographic grains corresponds to what is suspected about the distribution of the cholinergic innervation. An example of this would be the hippocampal formation which receives a cholinergic input from the septal area (26,27).

A point should be made with regard to the limitations of the resolution of the light microscope. It is evident from Fig. 1 that the autoradiographic grains are in the caudate–putamen and not in the corpus callosum, a fiber bundle. They are in association with regions that contain synapses (striatum) rather than fiber bundles, at least grossly. Synapses and dendrites are not visible in light microscopic material and to obtain this level of resolution, an electron microscope must be utilized. However, some data can be obtained that is at least compatible with the view that the receptors are in association with synapses. In Fig. 1A, the neuronal perikarya in the caudate–putamen are evident. The region between the cell bodies, the neuropil, appears as a gray matter of even texture and color. This is the area where the synapses occur. After a quantitative analysis of autoradiographic grain densities in the caudate putamen, it was found that there were more than 12 times as many receptors between cell bodies as there were over cell bodies (26,27). This would be expected if the bulk of the receptors were associated with synapses.

3. *Histochemistry with Propylbenzilylcholine Mustard*

In the studies with QNB, the drug was injected systemically and conditions were selected for specific labeling. In a recent study with PBC, the binding to histologic sections was performed *in vitro* where it is possible to control the incubation conditions to a high degree (37). The procedure utilized was to place frozen sections of unfixed rat brain on gelatin-coated slides and gently fix the tissue with 0.1% glutaraldehyde. After a preincubation step (some tissue with 10^{-6} M atropine for controls), low concentrations of high specific activity [^{3}H]PBC were added. The excess and unbound PBC was washed away and the tissue was postfixed, dipped in emulsion, and developed. Utilizing this procedure, Rotter et al. (37) were able to show rather dramatic localizations of muscarinic receptors to motor nuclei in the rat brainstem, particularly the hypoglossal nucleus. In other brain areas, Rotter et al. (37) found results similar to those of Kuhar and Yamamura (26,27), who utilized QNB. The PBC was localized throughout the neuropil of the hypoglossal nucleus. The cytoplasm and the nuclei of the large neurons in this nucleus were unlabeled.

Since PBC is irreversibly bound to the receptor, it was possible to expose the tissue with ligand bound to various "traumatic" conditions, that is, fixation and emulsion coating. It is questionable whether or not [^{3}H]QNB, a ligand that is reversibly bound, would have maintained a high degree of selective and unique localization to the receptor under these treatments. There probably would have been significant diffusion and loss of label and ligand from the tissue. Hence the ability to use irreversibly bound ligands rather than reversibly bound ones makes the experiments easier and more reliable for the investigator.

4. High Resolution Studies

To find out more precisely which membranes have the receptors, electron microscopic autoradiography must be utilized. At the time this chapter was written, such studies had not been published for the cholinergic muscarinic receptor. However the issues involved herein will be discussed to bring out some technical problems and to compare this situation with the previous light microscopic studies.

In preparing tissue for electron microscopy, one must embed the tissue to permit the cutting of ultrathin sections. This embedding procedure usually involves tissue fixation, dehydration, staining, and infiltration with the embedding agent and heating. Any one of these steps could have profound effects on the binding of a ligand to a receptor. Thus biochemical analyses must be performed at every stage of preparation for the electron microscope to be sure that artifacts are not introduced or that diffusion of ligand from receptor does not occur.

Can QNB be used as a ligand in electron microscopic studies? The difficulty is that [^{3}H]QNB is a reversible binding agent. It is quite possible that during the tissue processing, the dissociation rate of ligand would be enhanced and one might get a significant amount of diffusion of ligand from its receptor site. Diffusion that could be insignificant by light microscopic standards could seriously obliterate all meaningful information in electron microscopic studies.

Can [^{3}H]PBC be used as a ligand for electron microscopic studies? As in situations where QNB is used, it is possible to obtain a high degree of specific binding. A significant advantage is that it is bound irreversibly to the receptor. However, as mentioned above, electron microscopic results have not yet been reported and the experiments remain to be performed.

B. Cholinergic Nicotinic Receptors

It is now generally accepted that certain snake venoms bind very tightly, probably irreversibly, to cholinergic nicotinic receptors at the neuromuscular junction. A venom from *Bungarus multicinctus*, α-bungaratoxin (α-BGT), has been used in a number of studies. The evidence that α-BGT totally and irreversibly blocks the receptor is as follows: acetylcholine, acetylcholine analogs, and cholinergic nicotinic antagonists compete with α-BGT for receptor. In addition, the location of the binding sites in denervated muscle correlates well with the level of acetylcholine sensitivity. The venom binds selectively to cells with cholinergic nicotinic receptors, such as skeletal muscle, and does not bind elsewhere, such as to heart and fibroblast tissues (10,11,16,30,32). Because of the possibility of obtaining and preparing high specific activity ^{125}I-α-BGT, it is possible to perform a variety of autoradiographic studies on the localization of the cholinergic nicotinic receptors.

1. Light Microscopic Studies

In the light microscopic studies, it is possible to localize the cholinergic receptor binding to areas that are both acetylcholine-sensitive by electrophysiologic methods and rich in acetylcholinesterase, reflections of cholinergic innervation

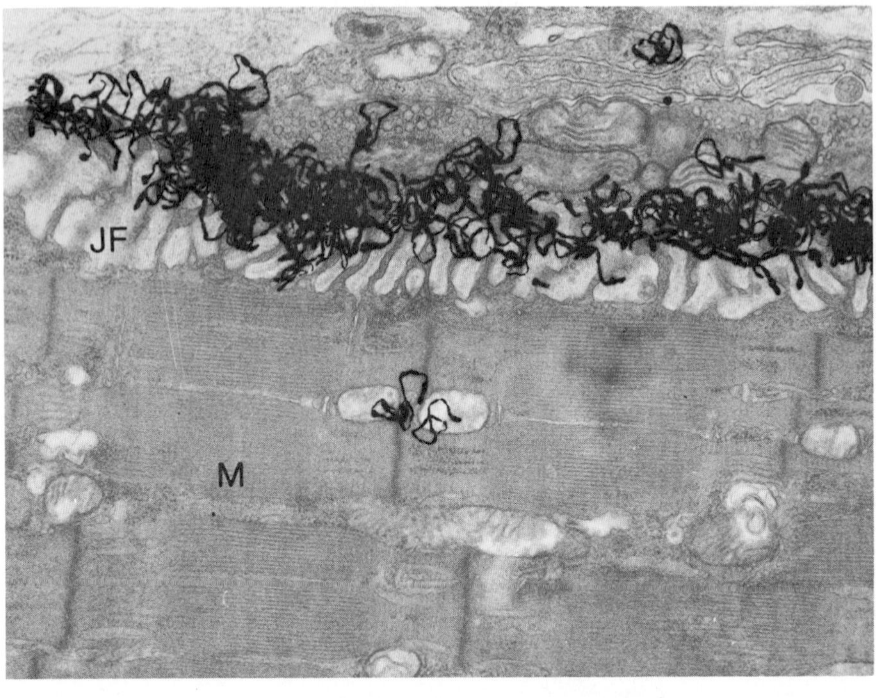

FIG. 2. Electron microscopic autoradiogram (Ilford L4 emulsion) of endplate from mouse sternomastoid muscle incubated with ^{125}I-labeled α-bungarotoxin until all neurally evoked muscle contractions were blocked. The autoradiogram is overexposed (i.e., the emulsion saturated with developed grains) in order to dramatize the illustration that the label is not uniformly distributed throughout the postjunctional membrane but is concentrated near the axonal interface. (JF) Junctional folds. (M) Muscle. ×18,900. (From Fertuck and Salpeter, ref. 19.)

(4,16,38). It has also been possible to perform a number of studies on the metabolism of receptor molecules themselves on muscle fibers in culture (14,15,33) as well as studies of the nicotinic receptor in disease (17) and development (22). Fluorescent conjugates of α-BGT have also been used in histochemical studies (25).

2. Electron Microscopic Studies

Electron microscopic studies of radiolabeled snake venom have been conducted. These have included α-BGT as well as the α-toxin purified from the venom of *Naja Nigricollis* (7,8,19). In these studies, because of the greater resolution of the electron microscope, it has been possible to study the localization of the receptor in greater detail. For example, α-BGT from *Naja Nigricollis* binds exclusively to the postsynaptic membrane of the electroplax organ of the electrical eel (7,8). In sternomastoid muscles of mice treated with radiolabeled α-BGT,

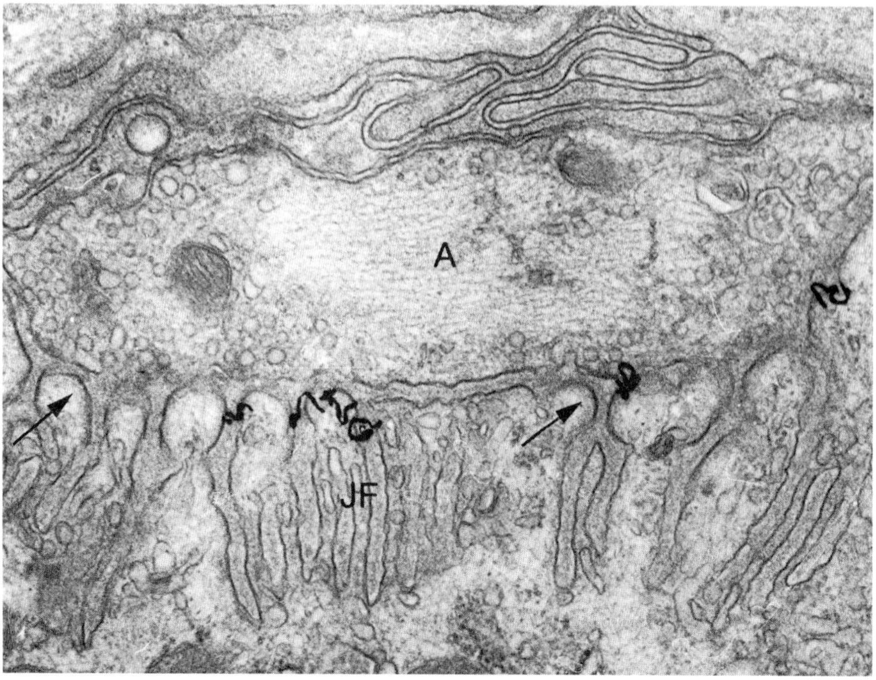

FIG. 3. Electron microscope autoradiogram of endplate labeled as in Fig. 2, but coated with the higher resolution emulsion Kodak NTE and not overexposed. Note the subneural location of the developed grains, again concentrated at the postjunctional membrane nearest the primary cleft and not distributed throughout the folds. ×33,750. (S) Schwann cell. (JF) Junctional folds. (A) Axon. (From Fertuck and Salpeter, ref. 19.)

receptors are found at the top of junctional folds, that is, at the postjunctional membrane nearest the axon (19). These results were obtained under conditions where α-BGT binding had eliminated the physiological muscle response. An example of some of these results are shown in Figs. 2 and 3. Thus by using a high-resolution method, it is clear that nicotinic receptors are not uniformly distributed throughout the synaptic area, but rather are concentrated near the axonal membrane. These results have important implications for studying and quantitating various aspects of neuromuscular transmission.

IV. SUMMARY

Histochemical methods are powerful tools in the study of neurotransmitter receptors. The basic techniques involve visualizing ligands bound to receptors. Thus the methods are indirect; that is, the ligands rather than the receptors are localized. Because of this, it is necessary to (a) selectively label receptors or have a way to determine which ligands are receptor-bound as opposed to nonspecifically bound and (b) be sure that the selective association of ligand and receptor is maintained throughout the histochemical procedures. A variety of techniques such as autoradiography and immunohistochemistry are feasible. In addition to light microscopic studies, high resolution studies with the electron microscope are feasible provided diffusion of ligand is eliminated. Even though the histochemistry of receptors is not an extensively developed area, several published experiments indicate that these methods can be used very successfully.

ACKNOWLEDGMENT

The author is the recipient of RSDA Award MH 00053 and acknowledges the excellent clerical assistance of Victoria Rhodes and Barbara Spink.

V. REFERENCES

1. Atweh, S. F., and Kuhar, M. J. (1977): Autoradiographic localization of opiate receptors in rat brain. I. Spinal cord and lower medulla. *Brain Res.,* 124:53–68.
2. Atweh, S. F., and Kuhar, M. J. (1977): Autoradiographic localization of opiate receptors in rat brain. II. The brainstem. *Brain Res.,* 129:1–12.
3. Atweh, S. F., and Kuhar, M. J. (1977): Autoradiographic localization of opiate receptors in rat brain. III. The telencephalon. *Brain Res.,* 134:393–405.
4. Barnard, E. A., Wieckowski, J., and Chiu, T. H. (1971): Cholinergic receptor molecules and cholinesterase molecules at mouse skeletal muscle junctions. *Nature (Lond.),* 234:207–209.
5. Beld, A. J., and Ariens, E. J. (1974): Stereospecific binding as a tool in attempts to localize and isolate muscarinic receptors. *Eur. J. Pharmacol.,* 25:203–209.
6. Bloom, F. E., Hoffer, B. J., Battenberg, E. F., Siggins, G. R., Steiner, A. L., Parker, C. W., and Wedner, H. J. (1972): Adenosine 3′,5′-monophosphate is localized in cerebellar neurons: Immunofluorescence evidence. *Science,* 177:436–438.
7. Bourgeois, J. P., Popot, J. L., Ryter, A., and Changeux, J. P. (1973): Consequences of denervation on the distribution of the cholinergic (nicotinic) receptor sites from Electrophorous electricus revealed by high resolution autoradiography. *Brain Res.,* 62:557–563.
8. Bourgeois, J. P., Ryter, A., Meney, A., Fromaglot, P., Boquet, P., and Changeux, J. P. (1972):

Localization of the cholinergic receptor protein in Electrophorus electroplax by high resolution autoradiography. *FEBS Lett.,* 25:127–133.
9. Burgen, A. S. V., Hiley, C. R., and Young, J. M. (1974): The binding of ^{3}H-propylbenzilylcholine mustard by longitudinal muscle strips from guinea pig small intestine. *Br. J. Pharmacol.,* 50:145–151.
10. Chang, C. C., and Lee, C. Y. (1963): Isolation of neurotoxins from the venom of Bungarus multicinctis and their modes of neuromuscular blocking action. *Arch. Int. Pharmacodyn.,* 144:241–257.
11. Changeux, J. P., Kasai, M., and Lee, C. Y. (1970): Use of a snake venom to characterize the cholinergic receptor protein. *Proc. Natl. Acad. Sci. USA,* 67:1241–1247.
12. Coons, A. H. (1958): Fluorescent antibody methods. In: *General Cytochemical Methods,* edited by J. F. Danielli, pp. 399–422. Academic Press, New York.
13. Creese, I., Burt, D. R., and Snyder, S. H. (1976): Dopamine receptor binding predicts clinical and pharmacological potencies of anti-schizophrenic drugs. *Science,* 192:481–483.
14. Devreotes, P. N., and Fambrough, D. M. (1975): Acetylcholine receptor turnover in membrane of developing muscle fibers. *J. Cell Biol.,* 65:335–358.
15. Devreotes, P. N., Gardner, J. M., and Fambrough, D. M. (1977): Kinetics of biosynthesis of acetylcholine receptor and subsequent incorporation into plasma membrane of cultured chick skeletal muscle. *Cell,* 10:365–373.
16. Fambrough, D. M., and Hartzell, H. C. (1972): Acetylcholine receptors: Number and distribution at neuromuscular junctions in rat diaphragm. *Science,* 176:189–191.
17. Fambrough, D. M., Drachman, D. B., and Satyamurti, S. (1973): Neuromuscular junction in myasthenia gravis: Decreased acetylcholine receptors. *Science,* 182:293–295.
18. Farrow, J. T., and O'Brien, R. D. (1974): Binding of atropine and muscarone to rat brain fractions and its relation to the acetylcholine receptor. *Mol. Pharmacol.,* 9:33–40.
19. Fertuck, H. C., and Salpeter, M. M. (1974): Localization of acetylcholine receptor by I^{125}-labeled α-bungarotoxin binding at mouse motor endplates. *Proc. Natl. Acad. Sci. USA,* 71:1376–1378.
20. Fields, J. Z., Reisine, T. D., and Yamamura, H. I. (1977): Biochemical demonstration of dopaminergic receptors in rat and human brain using ^{3}H-spiroperidol. *Brain Res.,* 136:578–584.
21. Goldman, M. (1968): *Fluorescent Antibody Methods.* Academic Press, New York.
22. Hartzell, N. C., and Fambrough, D. M. (1973): Acetylcholine receptor production and incorporation into membrane of developing muscle fibers. *Exp. Biol.,* 30:153–165.
23. Höllt, V., Cztonkowski, A., and Herz, A. (1977): The demonstration in vivo of specific binding sites for neuroleptic drugs in mouse brain. *Brain Res.,* 130:176–183.
24. Kebabian, J. W., Bloom, F. E., Steiner, A. L., and Greengard, P. (1975): Neurotransmitters increase cyclic nucleotides in postganglionic neurons: Immunocytochemical demonstration. *Science,* 190:157–158.
25. Ko, P. K., Anderson, M. J., and Cohen, M. W. (1977): Denervated skeletal muscle fibers develop discrete patches of high acetylcholine receptor density. *Science,* 196:540–542.
26. Kuhar, M. J., and Yamamura, H. I. (1975): Light autoradiographic localization of cholinergic muscarinic receptors in rat brain by specific binding of a potent antagonist. *Nature (Lond),* 253:560–561.
27. Kuhar, M. J., and Yamamura, H. I. (1976): Localization of cholinergic muscarinic receptors in rat brain by light microscopic radioautography. *Brain. Res.,* 110:229–243.
28. Kuhar, M. J., Murrin, L. C. Malouf, A., and Klemm, N. (1978): Dopamine receptor binding in vivo: The feasibility of autoradiographic studies. *Life Sci.,* 22:203–210.
29. Laduron, P., and Leysen, J. (1977): Specific in vivo binding of neuroleptic drugs in rat brain. *Biochem. Pharmacol.,* 26:1003–1007.
30. Lee, C. Y., and Chang, C. C. (1966): *Mem. Inst. Butantan,* 33:555.
31. Melamed, E., Lahau, M., and Atlas, D. (1976): Direct localization of β-adrenoceptor sites in rat cerebellum by a new fluorescent analogue of propranolol. *Nature (Lond),* 261:420–422.
32. Miledi, R., Molinoff, P., and Potter, L. T. (1971): Isolation of the cholinergic receptor protein of Torpedo electric tissue. *Nature (Lond),* 229:554–557.
33. Patrick, J., McMillan, J., Wolfson, H., and O'Brien, J. G. (1977): Acetylcholine receptor metabolism in a non-fusing muscle cell line. *J. Biol. Chem.,* 252:2143–2153.
34. Pert, C. B., Kuhar, M. J., and Snyder, S. H. (1975): Autoradiographic localization of the opiate receptor in rat brain. *Life Sci.,* 16:1849–1854.

35. Rogers, A. W. (1973): *Techniques of Autoradiography.* Elsevier, Amsterdam.
36. Roth, L. J., and Stumpf, W. E. (1969): *Autoradiography of Diffusible Substances.* Academic Press, New York.
37. Rotter, A., Birdsall, N. J. M., Burgen, A. S. V., Field, P. M., and Raisman, G. (1977): Axotomy causes a loss of muscarinic receptors and loss of synaptic contacts in the hypoglossal nucleus. *Nature (Lond),* 266:734–735.
38. Salpeter, M. M., and Eldefrawi, M. E. (1973): Sizes of endplate compartment densities of acetylcholine receptor and other quantitative aspects of neuromuscular transmission. *J. Histochem. Cytochem.,* 21:769–778.
39. Schubert, P., Höllt, V., and Herz, A. (1975): Autoradiographic evaluation of the intracerebral distribution of ^{3}H-etorphine in mouse brain. *Life Sci.,* 16:1855–1856.
40. Simon, E. J., Hiller, J. M., and Edelmann, I. (1973): Stereospecific binding of the potent narcotic analgesic (^{3}H)-etorphine to rat brain homogenate. *Proc. Natl. Acad. Sci. USA,* 70:1947–1949.
41. Speth, R. C., Chen, F. M., Lindstrom, J. M., Kobayashi, R. M., and Yamamura, H. I. (1977): Nicotinic cholinergic receptors in rat brain identified by [^{125}I] Naja, naja, siamensis α-toxin binding. *Brain Res.,* 131:350–355.
42. Stumpf, W. E., and Roth, L. G. (1966): High resolution autoradiography with dry mounted, freeze-dried frozen sections: Comparative study of six methods using two diffusable compounds, ^{3}H-estradiol and ^{3}H-mesobilirubinogen. *J. Histochem. Cytochem.,* 14:274–287.
43. Yamamura, H. I., and Snyder, S. H. (1974): Muscarinic cholinergic binding in rat brain. *Proc. Natl. Acad. Sci. USA,* 71:1725–1729.
44. Yamamura, H. I., Kuhar, M. J., and Snyder, S. H. (1974): In vivo identification of muscarinic cholinergic receptor binding in rat brain. *Brain Res.,* 80:170–176.

Neurotransmitter Receptor Binding, edited by
H. I. Yamamura et al.
Raven Press, New York © 1978.

7

Radioreceptor Assay Techniques for Neurotransmitters and Drugs

S. J. Enna

Departments of Pharmacology, Neurobiology, and Anatomy, The University of Texas Medical School at Houston, Houston, Texas 77025

I. INTRODUCTION

Many of the most significant advances made in understanding the chemical nature of neurotransmission and the biochemical mechanisms of drug action have resulted from the development of increasingly sensitive and sophisticated analytical procedures. For example, measurement of neurotransmitters has progressed from biological assays (35) and fluorometric techniques (27,29) to enzymatic–isotope methods (25,30) and gas chromatography–mass spectrometry (1); the major advantage of the newer techniques is their greater sensitivity. Thus picomole quantities of neurotransmitters can now be measured, making it possible to determine the concentration of these agents in discrete areas of the nervous system (17) and in biological fluids, such as cerebrospinal fluid (CSF) (37) and blood (16).

Ideally, an analytical method for measuring substances should be sensitive enough to measure biologically relevant quantities of the compound, specific only for the substance for which it is intended and simple enough to allow for the analysis of several samples at one time without extensive preparative procedures and expensive analytical equipment. One analytical procedure that fulfills these criteria is the analysis of substances by means of receptor-binding assays. The principle of these assays is based on the fact that the amount of radioactive substance specifically bound to a receptor site is a quantitative function of the amount of unlabeled substance present. Thus by simply performing a receptor binding assay in the presence of an unknown quantity of a substance that will interfere with the ligand binding to the receptor, the amount of substance can be calculated by determining the percent inhibition of radioligand binding and comparing this to the percent inhibition by known quantities of unlabeled ligand.

Probably the first practical use of this simple analytical procedure was suggested by Berson, Yalow, and colleagues (6) and utilized by this group (5) in their measurement of rabbit serum insulin levels by determining the amount of ^{131}I-insulin displaced from insulin-binding antibodies in the presence of serum. This type of assay is called a radioimmunoassay since it is based on the displacement of a radioactive antigen from a specific antibody. Since these early studies, radioimmunoassays for a number of immunologically active substances have been developed (21).

In contrast to radioimmunoassay, the radioligand-membrane receptor technique utilizes ligand binding to hormone and neurotransmitter receptor sites rather than an antigen–antibody reaction. This type of assay was first reported by Lefkowitz et al. (19), who demonstrated that the amount of unlabeled ACTH in a solution could be measured by determining the amount of ^{125}I-ACTH specifically bound to extracts of adrenal cortical tissue in the presence of the solution containing the unlabeled hormone. As a result of this development, techniques to measure numerous hormones and other substances such as cyclic AMP have been developed using radioligand receptor assay systems (15,18).

With the recent development of binding assays to study neurotransmitter receptors in the central nervous system (CNS), it is now possible to apply the same principles used for radioimmunoassays and radioligand–membrane receptor assays to study levels of neurotransmitters and drugs using the brain receptor-binding assay procedure. For the purposes of the present communication, the term radioreceptor assay will be used solely to refer to assays of neurotransmitters and drugs using CNS receptor-binding techniques, although this term can apply to radioimmunoassays and radioligand–membrane receptor assays as well. The development of these radioreceptor assays makes it possible for neuroscientists to rapidly, inexpensively, and accurately measure trace quantities of neurotransmitters and drugs in biological tissues and fluids and in some cases has allowed for the determination of substances that were impossible to measure accurately using standard procedures.

II. PRINCIPLES AND METHODOLOGY

A. Basic Principles

As with other competitive binding assays, the principle of the radioreceptor assay is based on the fact that the amount of radioactive ligand bound to brain membrane receptors is quantitatively related to the amount of unlabeled ligand present in the incubation medium. Thus at a fixed radioligand concentration the amount of specifically bound isotope will depend on the amount and affinity of unlabeled substance present in the incubation medium. As described in Chapters 2 and 4, the concentration of unlabeled ligand that will inhibit 50% of the radioligand binding will be roughly equivalent to the affinity constant of the unlabeled ligand for the receptor. Accordingly, the higher the affinity of the ligand for the receptor, the smaller the amount that can be accurately measured.

The assay itself is conducted using the procedure established to study receptor binding for the particular ligand to be investigated (see Chapter 4). Using this procedure, a small portion of the sample to be analyzed is added to the incubation medium and the percent of specifically bound radioligand remaining in the presence of the sample is compared to the percent of radioligand remaining after the addition of known amounts of the substance that is being analyzed, revealing the amount of substance in the sample.

When utilizing neurotransmitter receptor binding for a radioreceptor assay, it is essential that the conditions found to be optimum for receptor binding be utilized during the assay procedure. Thus for radioreceptor assay the radioligand concentration should be below the high-affinity binding constant for the ligand to assure maximum sensitivity. Also, the incubation buffer, temperature, and time should be such that binding equilibrium has been reached during incubation in order to obtain an accurate and reproducible value. Since receptor binding is linear over a specified range of tissue concentrations, it is also essential that the amount of tissue used for a radioreceptor assay be within this linear binding range to insure a precise determination of unlabeled substance. In brief, all of the general principles of receptor binding that have been discussed extensively in previous chapters apply when using transmitter receptor binding as the basis for radioreceptor analysis.

The first use of this technique for measuring a neurotransmitter substance was the measurement of brain levels of γ-aminobutyric acid (GABA) using the GABA receptor binding assay (9). Since this GABA assay is typical of all radioreceptor assays it will be used as an example to demonstrate the fundamental procedure.

B. Description of GABA Assay

1. Membrane Preparation

To study GABA receptor binding, crude synaptic membranes are prepared from rat brain (10) and then frozen at $-10°C$ for at least 18 hr prior to use. For the assay, the frozen pellets are resuspended in 0.05 M Tris-citrate buffer (pH 7.1 at 4° C) to a concentration of 1 mg protein/ml and sufficient Triton X-100 is added to yield a 0.05% final concentration of detergent. This suspension is incubated at 37° C for 30 min, then centrifuged at $48{,}000 \times g$ for 10 min. The resultant pellet is resuspended in a volume of water equivalent to the amount of buffer originally used, then centrifuged again as above. The pellet is resuspended in water and centrifuged a second time to rid the tissue of excess Triton, then resuspended a final time in 0.1 M Tris-citrate buffer. Freezing membranes and preincubating with 0.05% Triton X-100 enhances GABA receptor binding, yielding a more sensitive assay (11). The effect of these treatments seems to be peculiar for the GABA receptors and does not necessarily apply in other binding assays.

2. Sample Extraction

Conventional extraction procedures may be used to remove the substance to be analyzed from biological tissue. After extraction, and in some cases separation from other constituents in the initial extract that may interfere with binding, a small portion of the final extract is analyzed by means of the binding assay procedure.

For example, to measure endogenous GABA content of a brain sample, the sample is disrupted in water with a Polytron homogenizer and the homogenate centrifuged at $48{,}000 \times g$ for 10 min. Since GABA is a very water-soluble compound, virtually all of the brain GABA will be contained in the aqueous supernatant. A fraction of this supernatant is removed and diluted to the equivalent of 120 volumes with water and 20-μl portions of this solution are placed, in triplicate, into 16-ml Sorvall centrifuge tubes containing 1 ml of cold distilled water. The 120-fold dilution is made since previous tests had indicated that a dilution of this magnitude is necessary to have a GABA content in the analyzed sample that will displace between 20 and 70% of specifically bound [^{3}H]GABA. To the incubation tubes is then added 1 ml (0.3 to 0.8 mg protein), a range over which GABA binding is linear, of the crude synaptic membrane suspension and 20 μl of a [^{3}H]GABA (35 Ci/mmole) solution, which, in the 2-ml solution mixture, yields 8 nM [^{3}H]GABA (500,000 cpm) which is below the high affinity K_d for this receptor site. For maximum sensitivity it is essential that the radioligand concentration in the incubation medium be below the highest affinity K_d since displacement from this site will take the least amount of unlabeled ligand (see Chapters 2 and 4). After mixing, the samples are incubated at 4° C for 5 min and the reaction terminated by centrifugation at $48{,}000 \times g$ for 10 min.

For GABA binding a 5-min incubation time is used since GABA receptor binding is at equilibrium under these conditions. For all radioreceptor assays, it is essential to determine the percent displacement under equilibrium conditions in order to make an accurate determination of the potency of the unlabeled ligand. The time to reach equilibrium may vary from receptor to receptor. After centrifugation, the supernatant fluid is decanted and the pellet rinsed rapidly and superficially with 5 ml, then 10 ml, of ice cold distilled water. Membrane-bound radioactivity is extracted into a suitable tissue solubilizer, 10 ml of scintillation cocktail is added, and radioactivity assayed by liquid scintillation spectrometry. Total specific [^{3}H]GABA binding is obtained by subtracting from the total bound radioactivity the amount not displaced by 10^{-3} M unlabeled GABA or 10^{-4} M bicuculline, a GABA receptor antagonist. Using this procedure, total binding is approximately 8,000 cpm/mg protein and nonspecific binding (blank) is approximately 1,000 cpm/mg protein, yielding 7,000 cpm/mg protein specifically bound GABA. Again, the amount of specifically bound ligand will vary depending on the receptor assay being used as will the incubation time, buffer, and method of terminating the reaction. Thus it is essential that the proper conditions for receptor binding such as ligand and tissue concentration, incubation buffer, time, and temperature be established prior to using any particular receptor-binding procedure for a radioreceptor assay.

C. Generation of Standard Curve and Data Analysis

The amount of unlabeled ligand contained in a sample is simply calculated by determining the percent decrease in specifically bound radioligand observed in the presence of a known amount of extract and comparing this value to a standard curve of the radioligand displacement by known amounts of unlabeled ligand (Fig. 1). When plotted semilogarithmically, displacement curves for the inhibition of a radioactive ligand by unlabeled ligand yields a typical dose–response curve (Fig. 1A). Although this type of plot can be used as a standard curve, it is not entirely satisfactory since a significant percentage of it is nonlinear. However, data of this type can be converted to a linear dose–response curve by using logit paper (24), as illustrated for GABA receptor binding (Fig. 1B). Thus if 40% of the specifically bound [^{3}H]GABA was found remaining on membranes exposed to the brain extract, this would indicate the presence of 82 picomoles of GABA in the 20-μl extract samples.

Since, as discussed in previous chapters, the apparent affinity of a ligand for a receptor is dependent to a certain extent on the ligand and tissue concentration, and since these two factors may vary slightly from experiment to experiment, it is best to determine a standard curve for each experiment. For this purpose, four to five concentrations of standard that cover a range tenfold higher to tenfold lower than the affinity (K_d) of the ligand for the receptor should be sufficient.

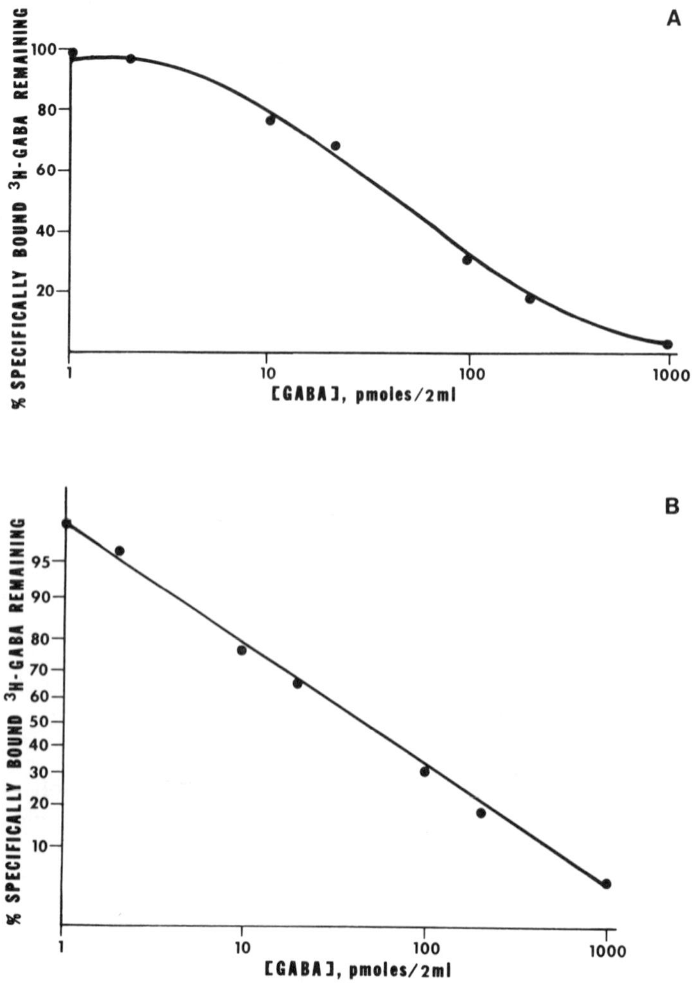

FIG. 1. Displacement of specifically bound [^{3}H]GABA from rat brain membranes by increasing concentrations of unlabeled GABA (see text for details). The data are plotted semilogarithmically **(A)** and after log-probit (logit) conversion **(B).**

As in all standard curves of this type, the most accurate portion is the middle of the displacement curve (30 to 70% remaining) since variability is greatest at the extremes. Accordingly, a dilution of the unknown should be made such that approximately 50% of the radioactive ligand will be displaced to insure the most accurate and precise determination.

It is also important to determine whether or not the vehicle containing the substance to be analyzed has any effect on specific ligand binding. For example, for some ligands, certain concentrations of salts may nonspecifically inhibit specific ligand binding such that analysis of the substance in a salt solution may lead to an erroneous value. Thus it is essential to determine what effect the concentration of solvent to be used in the assay will have on specific binding. For most radioreceptor assays this problem can be avoided by using a portion of the unknown sample that is 100 times or less the final incubation volume. A dilution of this magnitude will normally render most solvents inactive as nonspecific displacers.

It is also possible when analyzing substances dissolved in protein-containing solutions such as serum that there may be an increase in the binding blank since some of the radioactive ligand may bind nonspecifically to the serum protein. Obviously an increase in blank will also lead to an erroneous estimate of the concentration of the substance to be analyzed. Thus solvents containing organic material should also be analyzed for their ability to alter the amount of specifically bound isotope. Once again, however, a 100-fold or greater dilution in the assay will normally obviate this problem.

III. SENSITIVITY AND PRECISION

For radioreceptor assays, the lower limit of sensitivity is usually defined as that amount of substance that will displace 20% of the radioligand. This arbitrary figure is selected because the variability observed with displacement of less than 20% is too great to obtain a consistent determination.

Using [^{3}H]GABA with a specific activity of 35 Ci/mmole, the lower limit of sensitivity of the radioreceptor assay for GABA is 10 picomoles if a final incubation volume of 2 ml is used (Fig. 1B and Fig. 2). However, this sensitivity can be increased even further by decreasing the incubation volume (Fig. 2) and by decreasing the amount of tissue and radioligand proportionally to maintain an equivalent concentration. The reason for this increase in sensitivity with decreasing incubation volumes is that although the concentration that is necessary to displace 20% of the specifically bound ligand remains the same, the number of moles necessary to reach that concentration decreases as the volume decreases. For GABA, an unlabeled GABA concentration of approximately 50 nM will displace 20% of the specifically bound [^{3}H]GABA which, in a 20-ml incubation volume, is equivalent to 100 picomoles of unlabeled GABA. However, this same 50 nM concentration in a 2-ml or a 0.2-ml incubation volume is equivalent to only 10 and 1 picomoles, respectively (Fig. 2), making the smallest incubation volume the most sensitive.

Numerous factors determine the smallest volume that can be used for any radioreceptor assay. Probably the most crucial is the specific activity of the radioligand. Since as the volume is decreased the amount of radioligand and tissue must also be decreased, if, at a given specific activity, there are 7,000 cpm specifically bound in a 2-ml incubation volume, there will be 700 cpm specifically bound if the volume is reduced to 0.2 ml and only 70 cpm bound in a volume of 0.02 ml. Obviously it would be very difficult to accurately determine precise displacement figures if the total specific binding is only 70 cpm.

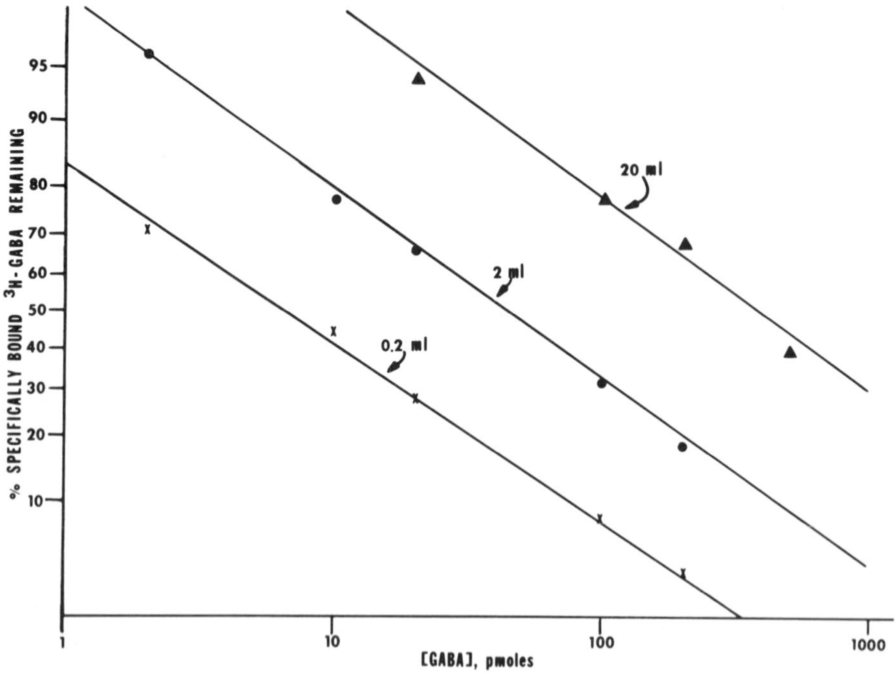

FIG. 2. Standard curves for displacement of specifically bound [^{3}H]GABA from rat brain membranes by unlabeled GABA using different incubation volumes (see text for details).

However, if the specific activity could be increased tenfold, then the assay sensitivity would also increase tenfold since now there would be 700 cpm bound in a 0.02-ml volume.

Another potential way to increase assay sensitivity is to find a radioligand having at least the same radiochemical specific activity as the commonly used ligand, but with a significantly higher affinity for the receptor site. For example, if, like [^{3}H]GABA, a radioligand has a specific activity of 35 Ci/mmole and an affinity for the receptor of 20 nM, then the lower limit of sensitivity would be approximately 1 pmole using a 0.2-ml incubation volume (Fig. 2). If, however, a radioligand is found that will specifically interact with the GABA receptor and also has a radiochemical specific activity of 35 Ci/mmole but has an affinity for the receptor of 2 nM, then, using this new radioligand, it would be possible to reduce the incubation volume to 0.02 ml and have the same number of counts bound as observed using a 0.2-ml incubation volume with [^{3}H]GABA, thereby increasing the sensitivity of the GABA assay tenfold. On the other hand, a ligand with a higher affinity for a receptor will not, in itself, be sufficient to increase the sensitivity of an assay if the specific activity of this new ligand is substantially less than the lower affinity ligand. Using the above example, if the new radioligand with an affinity of 2 nM has a specific activity of only 3

TABLE 1. *Estimated sensitivity of various receptor-binding procedures as radioreceptor assays*

Measurable substance	Radioligand	Incubation volume (ml)[a]	Lower limit of sensitivity[b] (pmole)	Ref.
GABA	[^{3}H]GABA	2	10	13
(−)-Norepinephrine	(−)-[^{3}H]Norepinephrine	1	5	34
(−)-Epinephrine	(−)-[^{3}H]Norepinephrine	1	1	34
Serotonin	[^{3}H]Serotonin	2	10	3
Dopamine	[^{3}H]Dopamine	1	5	7
Angiotensin II	[^{125}I]Angiotensin II	1	0.2	4
Neurotensin	[^{3}H]Neurotensin	1.25	0.5	33
Spiroperidol	[^{3}H]Spiroperidol	1	2	8
Diazepam	[^{3}H]Diazepam	2	2	20

[a] Incubation volume is the final volume used for assay.
[b] The estimated sensitivity is based on the amount of unlabeled substance which displaces 20% of the specifically bound radioligand.

Ci/mmole, then the assay sensitivity will not be increased at all since the number of counts bound in a 0.2-ml incubation volume will be similar to that observed for the ligand with ten times less affinity but a tenfold higher radiochemical specific activity. This is an important consideration since new, higher affinity ligands have been (2,14,31), and will continue to be, developed in the future. Accordingly, before attempting to use one of these new radioligands to improve the sensitivity of a radioreceptor assay, the specific activity relative to the increase in affinity must be taken into consideration.

Using 20% displacement as a lower limit, it is possible to estimate the sensitivity of various brain receptor-binding techniques as radioreceptor assays (Table 1). The lower limit of sensitivity listed for these assays was calculated by determining the amount of unlabeled ligand necessary to displace 20% of the specifically bound isotope. Thus with 1-ml incubation volumes or greater, all of these receptor-binding techniques can detect low picomole amounts of the indicated substances, demonstrating the exquisite sensitivity of the radioreceptor assay technique. In fact, because of the high specific activity of ^{125}I-angiotensin II, it would be quite possible to increase the sensitivity of this assay 20-fold using smaller volumes so that as little as ten femtomoles of angiotensin II could be readily detected.

With regard to precision, within an experiment, the percent of specifically bound isotope that is displaced by a particular concentration of unlabeled substance normally varies less than 5% among triplicate determinations. On the other hand, when the same sample is analyzed in different experiments the average variability is approximately 20%.

IV. SPECIFICITY

Since the radioreceptor assay is based on the displacement of specifically bound radioligand, any substance that has some affinity for the occupied receptor site will displace the isotope. This is the chief limitation of this analytical procedure. Thus before a brain receptor-binding technique can be utilized as a radioreceptor assay for any particular substance derived from any particular tissue or fluid, it is absolutely essential to demonstrate that the only substance in that tissue or fluid that will interfere with the radioligand binding is the substance that is being investigated. For example, if the norepinephrine concentration in adrenal medullary tissue was to be determined using a radioreceptor assay based on the receptor-binding technique listed in Table 1 for this compound, then it would not be possible to simply extract catecholamines from the tissue and analyze this extract due to the significant amount of epinephrine also present in this tissue which will also displace the specifically bound (−)[^{3}H]norepinephrine. Thus a step would have to be incorporated into the procedure to separate the two catecholamines before assay. A more subtle example of this concept is the effect of drugs on ligand binding. Thus brain serotonin can readily be determined using the [^{3}H]serotonin receptor assay technique but numerous drugs such as LSD, ergot alkaloids, and neuroleptics will also interfere with [^{3}H]serotonin binding if present in high enough concentrations. Accordingly, it must be demonstrated that the brain level of these substances does not interfere with [^{3}H]serotonin binding before the radioreceptor assay could be used to measure serotonin levels in animals treated with these substances.

Before using a radioreceptor assay to measure neurotransmitter or drug levels in biological tissues or fluids, it is also essential to present evidence that no naturally occurring substance in the fluid or tissue extract will interfere with binding. For example, the radioreceptor assay for GABA has now been used to measure the small quantities of this amino acid present in cerebrospinal fluid (12,13,36). For this assay, 200-μl portions of untreated CSF are placed into the incubation tubes containing the brain membranes and [^{3}H]GABA and the amount of GABA in the CSF is calculated by determining the amount of [^{3}H]GABA bound in the presence of the CSF sample. Preliminary displacement data revealed the presence of a substance or substances in CSF that was equivalent to approximately 200 picomoles of GABA per milliliter CSF. However, before it could be assumed that this displacing substance was GABA, other tests had to be performed to indicate that CSF does not contain some unknown compound that will also displace the specifically bound GABA. Subsequent qualitative and quantitative analysis did indeed demonstrate that the displacing substance in CSF is solely GABA indicating that the radioreceptor assay can be used to measure this amino acid in this fluid (12,13).

Since the binding of radioactive ligands to brain receptors is, by definition, specific, there are only a limited number of agents that will interfere with this process. In some cases however, even if a sample contains some substance other than the desired compound that will interact with the receptor-binding procedure, it may be possible to use a radioreceptor assay for analysis without separating the two constituents if the affinity and the concentration of the undesirable substance is such that it will not displace the ligand under the conditions of the experiment. Thus, imidazoleacetic acid is a metabolite of histamine that will displace specifically bound [^{3}H]GABA from the GABA receptor. It is possible that there is some imidazoleacetic acid in CSF, but the fact that this compound is significantly less potent than GABA in displacing [^{3}H]GABA and that the quantity of this substance in CSF is quite low explains why imidazoleacetic acid does not interfere with the analysis of CSF GABA using the radioreceptor assay.

V. OTHER APPLICATIONS

Radioreceptor assay techniques are useful in a number of situations where other procedures cannot be used or are too cumbersome or expensive. One example of this is the previously mentioned assay for GABA in CSF. Prior to using the radioreceptor assay, the only feasible methods for measuring the minute quantity of GABA in CSF were by gas chromatography–mass spectrometry (12) or ion exchange–fluorimetry (36). Although these methods are both sensitive and accurate for this purpose, both involve the use of expensive equipment and only a few samples can be analyzed at a time. With the radioreceptor assay, only routine biochemical reagents and equipment are used and as many as 200 samples can be analyzed in a day.

Another way in which radioreceptor assays have been used is to measure blood levels of neuroleptics and their metabolites (8). The development of this procedure represents a major breakthrough in the clinical management of patients taking these drugs since previous assays did not lend themselves to routine clinical use.

Radioreceptor assays have also been developed to rapidly and accurately determine brain and CSF levels of opioid peptides (22,23,26,28,32). These reports exemplify another use for radioreceptor assays in that they can be utilized to search for as yet undiscovered neurotransmitter or neuromodulating agents. Thus if a specific drug receptor is found in brain and if this site cannot be identified as a receptor for any known neurotransmitter, then the possibility exists that the brain contains some endogenous substance that will interact with this drug receptor site. The search for such a substance is simplified by using a radioreceptor assay since it is necessary only to determine if brain extracts will inhibit the binding of the drug to the brain receptor. If a brain extract does inhibit the binding, then the radioreceptor assay can be used as a tool to measure the relative concentration of the displacing substance during purification procedures and of course can ultimately be used to routinely measure the agent once it is identified.

Thus because of their simplicity, sensitivity, and specificity, radioreceptor assays have made it possible for neuroscientists to study drug and neurotransmitter levels that were previously very difficult, if not impossible to measure. This ability to measure picomole quantities of important neurochemicals should lead to a better understanding of the functional activity of these agents in biological systems.

VI. SUMMARY

Ligand-binding techniques to study brain neurotransmitter receptor sites can be used as assay procedures for measuring neurotransmitter and drug levels in biological tissues and fluids. The principle of these radioreceptor assay procedures is based on the fact that the amount of radioligand bound to the membrane receptor is quantitatively reduced by the amount of unlabeled ligand present. The chief limitation of radioreceptor assays is their specificity since any substance having an appreciable affinity for the neurotransmitter receptor site will displace the specifically bound ligand. Thus before routinely using a radioreceptor assay, precautions must be taken to ensure that the only substance in the sample that will interfere with ligand binding is the substance being analyzed. Because of the high specific activity of neurotransmitter radioligands, the radioreceptor assay procedure is very sensitive, being able to readily detect picomole quantities of compound. Radioreceptor assays are also simple, inexpensive, and rapid in that hundreds of samples can be analyzed in a single day. Studies have been reported using radioreceptor assays as analytical tools indicating the versatility and usefulness of this procedure in neurochemical investigations.

ACKNOWLEDGMENTS

Preparation of this manuscript was facilitated by grants from the following sources: USPHS MH-29739, Pharmaceutical Manufacturers Association, The Huntington's Chorea Foundation, Eli Lilly and Merck Sharp and Dohme. I thank Ms. Barbara Block for her excellent secretarial assistance.

VII. REFERENCES

1. Abramson, F. P. (1974): Femtomole level of analysis of biogenic amines and amino acids using functional group mass spectrometry. *Anal. Biochem.,* 51:482–499.
2. Beaumont, K., Chilton, W. S., Yamamura, H. I., and Enna, S. J. (1978): Muscimol binding in rat brain: Association with synaptic GABA receptors. *Brain Res. (in press).*
3. Bennett, J. P., and Snyder, S. H. (1976): Serotonin and lysergic acid diethylamide binding in rat brain membranes: Relationship to postsynaptic receptors. *Mol. Pharmacol.,* 12:373–389.
4. Bennett, J. P., and Snyder, S. H. (1976): Angiotensin II binding to mammalian brain membranes. *J. Biol. Chem.,* 251:7423–7430.
5. Berson, S., and Yalow, R. (1958): Isotopic tracers in the study of diabetes. *Adv. Biol. Med. Phys.,* 6:349–430.
6. Berson, S., Yalow, R., Bauman, A., Rothschild, M., and Newerly, K. (1956): Insulin-I^{131} metabolism in human subjects: Demonstration of insulin binding globulin in the circulation of insulin treated subjects. *J. Clin. Invest.,* 35:170–190.
7. Burt, D. R., Enna, S. J., Creese, I., and Snyder, S. H. (1975): Dopamine receptor binding in the corpus striatum of mammalian brain. *Proc. Natl. Acad. Sci. USA,* 72:4655–4659.
8. Creese, I., and Snyder, S. H. (1977): A novel, simple and sensitive radioreceptor assay for antischizophrenic drugs in blood. *Nature (Lond),* 270:261–263.
9. Enna, S. J., and Snyder, S. H. (1976): A simple, sensitive and specific radioreceptor assay for endogenous GABA in brain tissue. *J. Neurochem.,* 26:221–224.
10. Enna, S. J., and Snyder, S. H. (1975): Properties of γ-aminobutyric acid (GABA) receptor binding in rat brain synaptic membrane fractions. *Brain Res.,* 100:81–97.

11. Enna, S. J., and Snyder, S. H. (1977): Influences of ions, enzymes and detergents on GABA receptor binding in synaptic membranes of rat brain. *Mol. Pharmacol.,* 13:442–453.
12. Enna, S. J., Stern, L., Wastek, G., and Yamamura, H. I. (1977): Cerebrospinal fluid GABA variations in neurological disorders. *Arch. Neurol.,* 34:683–685.
13. Enna, S. J., Wood, J. H., and Snyder, S. H. (1977): γ-Aminobutyric acid (GABA) in human cerebrospinal fluid: Radioreceptor assay. *J. Neurochem.,* 28:1121–1124.
14. Fields, J., Reisine, T. D., and Yamamura, H. I. (1977): Biochemical demonstration of dopaminergic receptors in rat and human brain using ^{3}H-spiroperidol. *Brain Res.,* 136:578–584.
15. Gilman, A. G. (1970): A protein binding assay for adenosine 3′:5′-cyclic monophosphate. *Proc. Natl. Acad. Sci. USA,* 67:305–312.
16. Henry, D., Starman, B., Johnson, D., and Williams, R. (1975): A sensitive radio-enzymatic assay for norepinephrine in tissue and plasma. *Life Sci.,* 16:375–384.
17. Jacobowitz, D., Roizen, M., Suttora, N., and Muth, E. (1975): A method for the discrete removal of a segment of the dorsal noradrenergic bundle and its application to analysis of catecholamines and dopamine-β-hydroxylase. *Brain Res.,* 98:377–382.
18. Korenman, S. G. (1970): Relation between estrogen inhibitory activity and binding to cytosol of rabbit and human uterus. *Endocrinology,* 87:1119–1123.
19. Lefkowitz, R., Roth, J., and Pastan, I. (1970): Radioreceptor assay of adrenocorticotropic hormone: New approach to assay of polypeptide hormones in plasma. *Science,* 170:633–635.
20. Mohler, H., and Okada, T. (1977): Benzodiazepine receptor: Demonstration in the central nervous system. *Science,* 198:849–851.
21. Odell, W., and Daughaday, W., editors (1971): *Principles of Competitive Protein-Binding Assays.* Lippincott, Philadelphia.
22. Pasternak, G., Goodman, R., and Snyder, S. H. (1975): An endogenous morphine-like factor in mammalian brain. *Life Sci.,* 16:1765–1769.
23. Pasternak, G., Simantov, R., and Snyder, S. H. (1976): Characterization of an endogenous morphine-like factor (enkaphalin) in mammalian brain. *Mol. Pharmacol.,* 12:504–513.
24. Robard, D., and Lewald, J. E. (1970): Computer analysis of radioligand assay and radioimmunoassay data. *Acta Endocrinol.* [*Suppl*], 147:79–103.
25. Saavedra, J., Brownstein, M., and Axelrod, J. (1973): A specific and sensitive enzymatic-isotope microassay for serotonin in tissue. *J. Pharmacol. Exp. Ther.,* 186:508–515.
26. Shibuya, J., Bowie, D., and Pert, C. (1977): Opiate receptor ligand in cerebrospinal fluid: A simple radioreceptor assay requiring no preliminary purification. *Proc. Soc. Neurosci.,* 3:460.
27. Shore, P. A., and Olin, J. S. (1958): Identification and chemical assay of norepinephrine in brain and other tissues. *J. Pharmacol. Exp. Ther.,* 122:295–300.
28. Simantov, R., Childers, S., and Snyder, S. H. (1977): Opioid peptides: Differentiation by radioimmunoassay and radioreceptor assay. *Brain Res.,* 135:358–367.
29. Snyder, S. H., Axelrod, J., and Zweig, M. (1965): A sensitive and specific fluorescence assay for tissue serotonin. *Biochem. Pharmacol.,* 14:831–835.
30. Snyder, S. H., Baldessarini, R., and Axelrod, J. (1966): A sensitive and specific enzymatic isotopic assay for tissue histamine. *J. Pharmacol. Exp. Ther.,* 153:544–549.
31. Speth, R. C., Wastek, G. J., Johnson, P. C., and Yamamura, H. I. (1978): Benzodiazepine binding in human brain: Characterization using ^{3}H-fluornitrazepam. *Life Sci.,* 22:859–866.
32. Terenius, L., and Wahlstrom, A. (1975): Search for an endogenous ligand for the opiate receptor. *Acta Physiol. Scand.,* 94:74–81.
33. Uhl, G. R., and Snyder, S. H. (1976): Regional and subcellular distribution of brain neurotensin. *Life Sci.,* 19:1827–1832.
34. U'Prichard, D. C., and Snyder, S. H. (1977): ^{3}H-Epinephrine and ^{3}H-norepinephrine binding to α-noradrenergic receptor in calf brain membranes. *Life Sci.,* 20:527–534.
35. VonEuler, U. S. (1947): A specific sympathomimetic ergone in adrenergic nerve fibers (sympathin) and its relations to adrenaline and noradrenaline. *Acta Physiol. Scand.,* 12:73–97.
36. Wood, J., Glaeser, B., Enna, S. J., and Hare, T. (1978): Verification and quantification of GABA in human CSF. *J. Neurochem.,* 30:291–293.
37. Ziegler, M., Lake, C., Foppen, F., Shoulson, I., and Kopin, I. (1976): Norepinephrine in cerebrospinal fluid. *Brain Res.,* 108:436–440.

Neurotransmitter Receptor Binding, edited by
H. I. Yamamura et al.
Raven Press, New York © 1978.

8

Receptor Binding as a Primary Drug Screening Device

Ian Creese

Department of Pharmacology and Experimental Therapeutics, Johns Hopkins University School of Medicine, Baltimore, Maryland 21205

I. INTRODUCTION

It is often stated that the major discoveries in drug therapy have been made by serendipity. This is obviously a truism when one considers the development of the ancient pharmacopoeias. There was generally no rational reason for choosing one herb over another for the treatment of a particular ailment. Often a morphological similarity between a plant and the desired result was sufficient to ensure its success. But must serendipity play such a pivotal role in modern drug development? The means by which neurotransmitter receptor methodology can provide a cornerstone in the rational development of new therapeutic agents will be described in this chapter.

A. Toward a Rational Approach to Drug Design

Modern pharmacology has been based on a more logical isomorphism. By taking an already proven therapeutic drug one can synthesize many new compounds of similar structure. Since chemists have an unlimited capability to produce novel compounds and since ethical considerations preclude the initial testing of new compounds in humans, this multitude of potential drugs is generally screened in animals. When considering drugs that have a peripheral locus of action, such animal models are very often satisfactory. Thus homology can be observed in the mechanisms by which histamine H_2-antagonists, anticancer agents, or antibiotics ameliorate duodenal ulcers, metastases, or bacterial infection in rats, monkeys, and man. However, in considering animal screens for psychotropic drugs with a central locus of action such obvious homology in mechanism or symptom is often absent. For example, the exact relationship between the mechanism by which a drug relieves a schizophrenic of auditory hallucinations and stops a rat from jumping up on a pole to avoid an electric shock (a common screen for antischizophrenic agents) is hard to discern. Such screens have been shown empirically to correlate with pharmacological potency in man. Whether or not there is a similar biochemical or physiological substrate for these, on the surface, dissimilar effects is generally unknown.

The enormous intake of psychotropic drugs in American society today implies a widespread acceptance of a mechanistic approach to mental well-being and illness by the pharmaceutical industry, medical profession, and general public at large. Working within this framework psychopharmacology has been remarkably successful by many criteria. Neuroleptics have emptied mental institutions, lithium and antidepressants have calmed and animated the manic–depressive, and minor tranquilizers such as diazepam have enabled many to cope with the increasing stress of modern society. However, there is room for much improvement. Almost all psychotropic drug therapy to date is prone to cause unwanted side effects. Significant numbers of patients do not respond to the drugs that are successful for other patients with a superficially similar symptomology, probably indicating subclasses within our rather broad general categories of mental illness, where different physiological processes are disturbed. Thus new drugs that are more potent, more specific, shorter or longer acting are needed, as well as novel compounds to treat the significant proportion of refractory patients who are not "possessed by evil spirits."

This mechanistic approach to mental illness and neurological disease implies a correlative disturbance in brain functioning and hence brain biochemistry. To date much of modern psychopharmacology has been based on the hypothesis that a single biochemical deficit may explain global mental and behavioral disturbances and thus be amenable to simple and rational biochemical therapy. If one works within such a framework two general approaches to rational drug design are possible: (a) determination of the exact biochemical mechanism of action of a known therapeutic agent and development of new compounds that are more specific, potent, and so forth, and (b) determination of the exact biochemical deficit responsible for the disease, and production of an identical biochemical lesion in animals and search, on a systematic basis, for drugs to counteract its effects.

B. Receptor-Binding Studies

Although there are many possible biochemical sites of action for a drug, electrophysiological, pharmacological, and behavioral studies have provided strong indications that many classes of psychotropic drugs probably act by binding to neurotransmitter receptors, either as agonists or antagonists. During the past 5 years neurotransmitter receptor-binding studies have provided a new method to screen for the biochemical mechanism of action of psychotropic drug activity *in vitro*. In the following sections we will discuss how various neurotransmitter receptor-binding studies can demonstrate the molecular mechanism of psychotropic drug action in producing their therapeutic effects. The characterization of the neurotransmitter receptor site through which a particular drug class produces its pharmacological effects thus provides an excellent *in vitro* drug-screening system for novel compounds. Specific examples from various psychotropic drug classes will form the framework for each section. Such receptor-binding/drug screens have many beneficial characteristics. They enable detailed structure-activity relationships to be examined unencumbered by variations in absorption or metabolism. This is obviously an efficient way in which to focus on the pharmacologically active portions of a molecule and direct further synthetic programs. With regard to the receptor recognition site, receptor-binding screens are unlikely to yield false positives or false negatives—if a drug binds with high affinity, then, all else being equal, it should be an active agonist or antagonist; if it does not bind, then it will not be active. In some cases by screening a compound on several receptors it is also feasible to determine its possible side effects. These screens are rapid, inexpensive, and require only milligram quantities of new compounds.

II. RECEPTOR STUDIES AS A SCREEN FOR MECHANISM OF DRUG ACTION

The molecular mechanism of action of a therapeutic drug may be suggested by the biochemical event that correlates best with clinical potency. Correlation, of course, does not prove causality. However, if a significant number of drugs are available that have been used clinically and, ranked according to molar potency, demonstrate a high correlation with their potency in a particular *in vitro* biochemical system, then such a causal relationship would be strongly suggested and warrant further study. Even if it were not possible to demonstrate directly a causal relationship, such an *in vitro* biochemical system could provide a satisfactory pragmatic screen for other compounds with similar activity that could then undergo clinical tests.

A. Neuroleptics

The interactions of neuroleptic drugs with neurotransmitter receptors will be discussed in great detail since binding studies have demonstrated that both the therapeutic effects of neuroleptics as well as their major side effects are probably mediated through neurotransmitter receptor interactions. To date these are probably the most researched receptor-binding drug screens and consequently they provide a good framework on which to design investigations of other drug receptor interactions.

Since the serendipitous discovery and introduction of chlorpromazine by Delay and Deniker in 1952 for the treatment of schizophrenia (14), a large number of phenothiazines of different potencies have been successfully introduced into clinical practice. That their therapeutic potency as antipsychotic agents was paralleled by their ability to sedate and induce catalepsy (a "waxy" rigidity) in rats suggested this as a useful animal screen for new compounds. The chance observation that a butyrophenone derivative of the opiate norpethidine also induced catalepsy and sedation led Janssen to synthesize more than 4,000 related compounds during the past 20 years (20). This massive synthetic program was certainly warranted for the butyrophenones, which are chemically quite distinct from the phenothiazines, but are very potent as antipsychotic agents.

Further pharmacological studies demonstrated that the phenothiazines and butyrophenones, although chemically diverse, shared the ability to antagonize amphetamine and apomorphine-induced behavior in animals. Since apomorphine is a dopamine analog and amphetamine can release dopamine from, and block its reuptake into, adrenergic presynaptic terminals, these results indicated that neuroleptic drugs blocked postsynaptic dopamine receptors. Carlsson had previously suggested this common mechanism of action for neuroleptics from studies of their effects on dopamine turnover (reviewed in ref. 8). The potency of various neuroleptics in these systems correlated with clinical potency, suggesting the unitary hypothesis that dopamine receptor blockade might mediate their antischizophrenic activity (22).

If the biochemical locus for the therapeutic action of a class of drugs has been correctly identified, then the concentration of drug required to interact with the system must be within the range of its determined *in vivo* level. The phenothiazine nucleus is highly reactive chemically and these drugs are very hydrophobic, surface-active substances that readily accumulate in cell membranes. Soon there were many reports of their influences on various enzyme or membrane properties (8). However, all these effects occurred in the μM–mM range, a concentration not likely to be obtained *in vivo*. Furthermore there was no correlation between the potencies of different drugs in producing these various effects and their antipsychotic activities.

The definitive demonstration that both phenothiazines and butyrophenones do indeed block dopamine receptors in proportion to their clinical antipsychotic efficacy came from dopamine receptor-binding studies. Initial studies labeled binding sites in calf striatum with the butyrophenone [^{3}H]haloperidol (4,32). Approximately 30% of [^{3}H]haloperidol binding was displaceable by physiological concentrations of dopamine, suggesting that it might be binding to dopamine receptors. However, haloperidol itself competed with [^{3}H]haloperidol in an atypical way, with continuous displacement over a very wide concentration range (Fig. 1). This indicated that [^{3}H]haloperidol, not surprisingly, was binding to a number of different sites with differing affinities (2).

A useful determinant for identifying the biochemical site of drug action is that of stereospecificity. If *in vivo* activity of a drug is exhibited only by one of its optical or geometric isomers, then such differences in isomeric activity must also be exhibited in the correct *in vitro* system. Butaclamol, a neuroleptic of the dibenzocycloheptane class, exists in the form of optical isomers. Only (+)—butaclamol exhibits dopamine-blocking activity *in vivo* in animal models and is antischizophrenic, whereas (−)—butaclamol is many hundred-fold less active. (+)—Butaclamol displays two clearly distinct components in inhibiting [^{3}H]haloperidol binding. The high-affinity component elicits half maximal effects at approximately 1 nM whereas the lower-affinity component is only apparent at concentrations above 1 μM (Fig. 1). In contrast, (−)—butaclamol lacks the high-affinity component of inhibition of [^{3}H]haloperidol binding whereas its lower-affinity inhibition of [^{3}H]haloperidol binding resembles the low-affinity influence of (+)—butaclamol. Physiological concentrations (1 to 100 μM) of dopamine maximally reduces [^{3}H]haloperidol binding to the same extent as the high-affinity component of (+)—butaclamol inhibition and these inhibitions are not additive.

The properties of this stereospecific butaclamol displaceable [^{3}H]haloperidol binding was further investigated to determine if it was indeed labeling dopamine receptors. In regard to agonist specificity, apomorphine, a dopamine analog

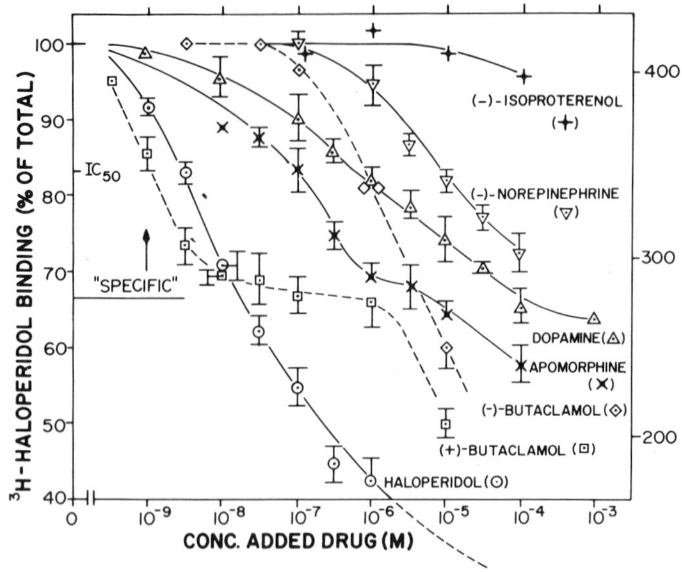

FIG. 1. Displacement of [^{3}H]haloperidol binding to calf striatal membranes by nonradioactive drugs. (From ref. 2.)

and an *in vivo* agonist, displayed a K_i of 50 nM. It was more potent than dopamine ($K_i = 670$ nM) which in turn was more potent than epinephrine and norepinephrine (K_i's approximately 5,000 nM). Other neurotransmitter and putative neurotransmitter agonists such as acetylcholine, serotonin, GABA, glycine, enkephalin, and isoproterenol were inactive (2). This indicated that [^{3}H]haloperidol was indeed labeling dopamine receptors. Regional studies indicated high levels of binding in caudate nucleus (approximately 20 picomoles per gram wet weight) with lower binding in the putamen and mesolimbic areas. No stereospecific butaclamol displaceable binding was detected in the cerebellum (2). These results mirrored the terminal innervations of the dopamine pathways.

Investigations of a large number of phenothiazine, butyrophenone, and related neuroleptic drugs (5,6,33) have demonstrated that there is an excellent correlation between the molar pharmacological potencies of these agents in animals and man and their affinities for [^{3}H]haloperidol-binding sites. For example, antagonism of apomorphine-induced stereotyped behavior in rats is a classic neuroleptic screen that generally predicts antischizophrenic potency. The affinities of the neuroleptics for [^{3}H]haloperidol-binding sites correlate highly with their molar potency in antagonism of apomorphine-induced stereotypy ($r = 0.94$, $p < 0.001$) (Fig. 2). There is also a highly significant correlation between neuroleptic affinity for dopamine receptor-binding sites and antagonism of amphetamine-induced stereotyped behavior in the rat ($r = 0.92$, $p < 0.001$). Similarly blockade of apomorphine-induced emesis in dogs correlates closely with [^{3}H]haloperidol-binding

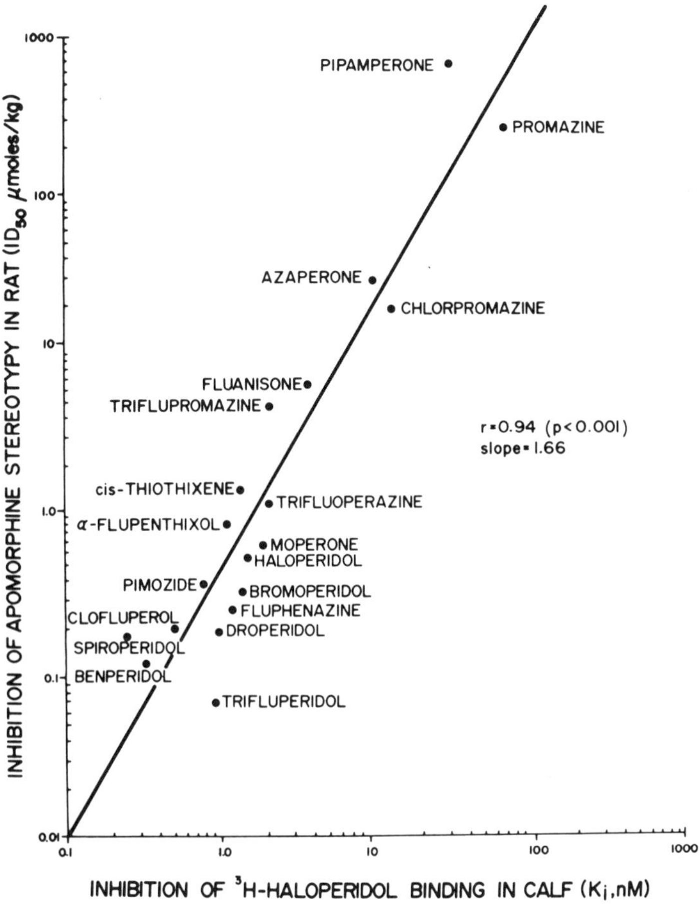

FIG. 2. Correlation of neuroleptic drug affinity for [^{3}H]haloperidol binding sites in calf striatal membranes and antagonism of apomorphine stereotypy in the rat. (From ref. 40.)

site affinity ($r = 0.93$, $p < 0.001$). This is one of the most sensitive *in vivo* neuroleptic assays and is presumed to involve the blockade of dopamine receptors in the vicinity of the chemoreceptor trigger zone in the brain stem where the blood–brain barrier may be less effective.

It seems likely that these results demonstrate that dopamine receptor blockade is responsible for the pharmacological effects of the neuroleptics in these animal screens since 16 or more drugs of quite varied chemical structure were examined in these correlations, suggesting that the results were probably not spurious or related to only one family of structures. Furthermore, drug potencies differed by more than 1,000-fold in both the *in vitro* and *in vivo* screens. It is important to note that when making such comparisons the milligram per kilogram *in vivo* dose should be converted to moles, free base per kilogram. These data also indicate that in these acute animal experiments drug metabolism, absorption, and penetration probably do not play a major role in determining differences in *in vivo* potency. Furthermore, these animal data (reviewed by Janssen and Van Bever, ref. 22) were determined objectively in controlled conditions using many animals to produce detailed dose–response curves. It is also dramatic that the clinical potency of these drugs as antipsychotic agents in man, simply determined by the average daily oral effective dose, also correlates very highly with competition for [^{3}H]haloperidol binding ($r = 0.87$, $p < 0.001$) (Fig. 3) (5). These impressive correlations indicate the affinity of a drug for the [^{3}H]haloperidol-binding site of dopamine receptors is a powerful predictor of *in vivo* dopamine receptor antagonism and antipsychotic activity. The nM affinity of these drugs for dopamine receptor-binding sites is also in line with the plasma concentrations of these drugs at therapeutic dose levels as measured by the neuroleptic radioreceptor assay (12) (see Chapter 7) and other methods.

It is important to point out that a poor correlation between *in vivo* and *in vitro* activities can occur even when investigating the correct biochemical site of action for a series of drugs. For example, among neuroleptic drugs, reserpine was one of the first to have been used clinically and it has a behavioral profile

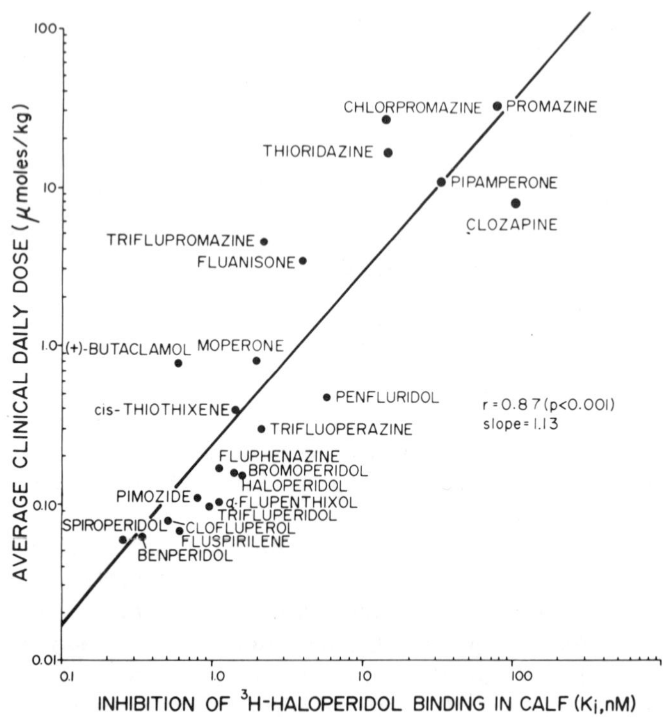

FIG. 3. Correlation of neuroleptic drug affinity for [^{3}H]haloperidol binding sites in calf striatal membranes and antipsychotic activity in man. (From ref. 6.)

similar to the phenothiazines and the butyrophenones. However, it has a very low affinity for the dopamine receptor (> 1 μM). In fact, reserpine does act via dopamine receptors but in an indirect fashion. It depletes dopamine stores in the presynaptic terminal, indirectly decreasing dopaminergic activity at the postsynaptic receptors. It is thus important to bear in mind that a single common biochemical (and therapeutic) outcome can occur via more than one mechanism. Correlations can also be disturbed because a therapeutic agent has its biochemical efficacy mediated by the activity of a potent metabolite produced *in vivo,* which is not produced during the *in vitro* binding assays.

The utility of this dopamine receptor-binding screen for neuroleptic drugs has been improved recently by the introduction of [^{3}H]spiroperidol as ligand. Specific [^{3}H]spiroperidol binding to the dopamine receptor accounts for 90% of total striatal [^{3}H]spiroperidol binding (11,18). As such this is a more robust assay and problems of multiple binding sites and additivity do not arise. The properties of [^{3}H]spiroperidol binding are, in essence, identical to those of [^{3}H]haloperidol in all other respects. Thus the selective high affinity of a novel compound for striatal [^{3}H]spiroperidol binding sites would be predictive of *in vivo* neuroleptic activity.

Although the stereospecific interaction of butaclamol with [^{3}H]haloperidol-binding sites suggested that these sites might be responsible for the therapeutic effects of neuroleptics, stereospecificity *per se* (without the confirmatory studies of large numbers of other neuroleptics) is a necessary but not sufficient criterion. For example, neuroleptics also manifest stereoselectivity in competing for [^{3}H]WB-4101 binding to the α-norepinephrine receptor. Among neuroleptics with geometric isomers, neuroleptic action in man and animals is manifested selectively by *cis*-thiothixene and α-flupenthixol but not by their *trans*- or β-isomers. In line with this, *cis*-thiothixene is approximately 100 times more potent than *trans*-thiothixene and α-flupenthixol is approximately 50 times more potent than β-flupenthixol in blocking [^{3}H]haloperidol binding. These isomeric differences are maintained, although to a substantially lesser extent, in inhibiting [^{3}H]WB–4101 binding where the active isomers of these drugs are 23-fold and 3.6-fold more potent, respectively. (+)—Butaclamol has an affinity of 35 nM for [^{3}H]WB–4101 binding and is 70 times more potent than its (−)—isomer (17). (+)—Butaclamol exhibits a greater than 1,000-fold stereoselectivity at [^{3}H]haloperidol-binding sites (2).

These results emphasize the fact that stereospecificity and correlations between clinical and biochemical effects must be critically examined before assuming a particular effect is the primary biochemical site of action. For example the stereospecific influences of neuroleptics on receptor binding for numerous ligands has been examined (16). Only the binding of [^{3}H]LSD and [^{3}H]serotonin is also inhibited stereospecifically and with considerable potency by these neuroleptics (Table 1). Thus (+)—butaclamol is 140 times as potent (IC_{50} 50 nM) as (−)—butaclamol in lowering [^{3}H]LSD binding. This neuroleptic is somewhat less potent in lowering the binding of [^{3}H]5-HT (1 μM) but still displays a

TABLE 1. *Displacement of various receptor ligands by neuroleptic isomers*

Compound	IC$_{50}$ (μM)										
	[^{3}H]DHA[a]	[^{3}H]5-HT[b]	[^{3}H]LSD[c]	[^{3}H]DA[d]	[^{3}H]Halo[e]	[^{3}H]QNB[f]	[^{3}H]Stry[g]	[^{3}H]Nal[h]	[^{3}H]DHM[i]	[^{3}H]GABA[j]	[^{3}H]WB[k]
(+)-Butaclamol	>100	1.0	0.05	0.1	0.001	100	>100	18	17	>100	0.035
(−)-Butaclamol	>100	8.0	7.0	16.0	1.3	40	>100	20	17	>100	2.5
α-Flupenthixol	>100	4.0	0.10	0.2	0.002	0.7	>100	55	100	100	0.007
β-Flupenthixol	>100	60.0	6.0	10.0	0.10	0.9	>100	50	100	>100	0.15
cis-Thiothixene	80	1.0	0.3	0.7	0.003	3.2	50	15	30	50	0.10
trans-Thiothixene	80	7.0	1.0	19.0	0.30	2.8	50	15	35	50	0.036

Adapted from ref. 16.

[a] Rat cerebral cortex membranes; [^{3}H]DHA = 1 nM, dihydroalprenolol.
[b] Rat cerebral cortex membranes; [^{3}H]5-HT = 7 nM, serotonin.
[c] Rat cerebral cortex membranes; [^{3}H]LSD = 3 nM, lysergic acid diethylamide.
[d] Calf striatal membranes; [^{3}H]DA = 5 nM, dopamine.
[e] Calf striatal membranes; [^{3}H]Halo = 2 nM, haloperidol.
[f] Rat forebrain homogenate; [^{3}H]QNB = 1 nM, quinuclidinyl benzilate.
[g] Rat spinal cord–brainstem, synaptosomal membranes; [^{3}H]Stry = 2 nM, strychnine.
[h] Rat forebrain membranes; [^{3}H]Nal = 1 nM, naloxone.
[i] Rat forebrain membranes; [^{3}H]DHM = 1 nM, dihydromorphine.
[j] Rat brain synaptosomal membranes; [^{3}H]GABA = 8 nM, γ-aminobutyric acid.
[k] Rat brain membranes; [^{3}H]WB-4101 = 0.22 nM.

degree of stereospecificity. However, since the neuroleptics are at least 50 times weaker at inhibiting [^{3}H]LSD binding than they are at inhibiting [^{3}H]haloperidol binding, in spite of these stereospecific effects, blockade of 5-HT receptors is probably not a major source of neuroleptic clinical efficacy. In addition, the relative influences of an extensive series of these drugs on [^{3}H]LSD binding does not correlate with clinical potency, further tending to support the notion that the serotonin receptor is not their primary site of action (1). Similarly, although the butyrophenones and related neuroleptics are reasonably active ($IC_{50} \sim 10$ μM) at inhibiting GABA uptake (16) or [^{3}H]naloxone binding to the opiate receptor (9) it is unlikely that either of these properties is the main determinant of their antischizophrenic activity. Their affinity is approximately 1,000-fold lower in these systems than at the dopamine receptor [^{3}H]haloperidol-binding site and when phenothiazine affinity for GABA uptake sites or opiate receptors is considered as well, there is a poor correlation with clinical efficacy (16).

B. Benzodiazepines

Recently, a selective receptor-binding assay for the benzodiazepines has become a reality. Mohler and Okada (26) and Squires and Braestrup (43) have identified [^{3}H]diazepam binding of high affinity to brain membranes. The affinity of these binding sites for diazepam is considerable with a K_D of approximately 3 nM. There is an excellent correlation between the affinity of numerous benzodiazepines for these binding sites and their *in vivo* potency in many animal screens, such as the cat muscle relaxant test ($r = 0.9$), predictive of anxiolytic action (Fig. 4). Moreover, these binding sites also exhibit stereospecificity, with the pharmacologically active isomer of optically isomeric benzodiazepines having highest affinity.

Are the benzodiazepines binding to a neurotransmitter receptor? No known neurotransmitter or putative neurotransmitter has substantial affinity for these binding sites. Neither do any other class of psychotropic drugs or neurotransmitter agonists or antagonists have marked influence on these binding sites. Strikingly, barbiturates, GABA, glycine, and strychnine are without effect on [^{3}H]diazepam binding. This may indicate that the binding sites mediate only the anxiolytic and muscle relaxant actions of the benzodiazepines and not their sedative effects. Regional studies give little clue to the precise locus for the pharmacological actions of the benzodiazepines since binding sites appear to be rather ubiquitous, with relatively moderate regional variations throughout the brain. Studies are under way in many laboratories that are an attempt to isolate from brain extracts "an endogenous ligand" for the benzodiazepine receptors.

Such experiments will obviously shed much light on the mechanism of action of benzodiazepines. But even without such knowledge it appears clear that the

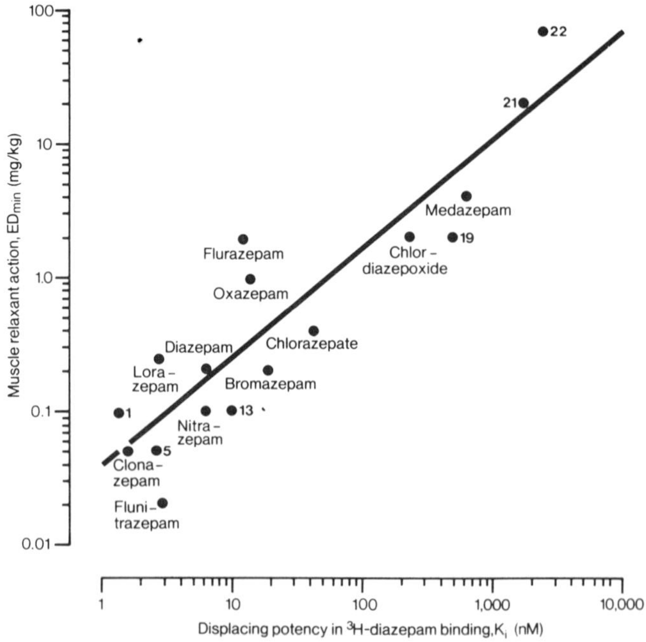

FIG. 4. Benzodiazepines: correlation between muscle relaxant effect and affinity for [^{3}H]diazepam-binding sites. Numbers on graph indicate RO code number: 1 = RO5-3027; 5 = -3590; 13 = -2904; 19 = -3636; 21 = -5807; and 22 = -4933. (Taken from ref. 26, copyright 1978 by the AAAS.)

[^{3}H]diazepam-binding assay can be used pragmatically as a screen for new drugs with specific anxiolytic and muscle relaxant effects.

In using correlation techniques to determine biochemical sites of action of therapeutic drugs, it is important to use quantitative data to compare *in vivo* and *in vitro* potencies. For example, [^{3}H]strychnine, a potent glycine antagonist, binds to synaptic membrane preparations of spinal cord and brain stem to a site probably associated with the ionophore of the glycine receptor (50). Of the many compounds studied, including barbiturates and other sedatives, only amino acids with glycine-like activity in electrophysiological studies and the benzodiazepines have marked affinity for [^{3}H]strychnine-binding sites (51).

In a series of 21 benzodiazepines examined there was a 50-fold variation in potency with regard to [^{3}H]strychnine displacement, with IC_{50} values ranging from 20 μM to 1 mM. Diazepam (IC_{50} 26 μM) was as potent as glycine in inhibiting [^{3}H]strychnine binding. Using rank order correlation techniques, significant correlations were observed between benzodiazepines' pharmacological actions and their affinities for [^{3}H]strychnine-binding sites (51). Significant correlations were found between glycine receptor affinity and human anxiolytic potency ($r = 0.74$) and in animal screens for anxiolytics such as the muscle relaxation test in the cat ($r=0.78$). Nonsignificant correlations were found between animal screens, such as continuous avoidance with escape failure ($r=0.16$), which are not predictive of anxiolytic activity.

Since barbiturates are inactive at inhibiting [^{3}H]strychnine binding it was hypothesized that the anxiolytic and muscle relaxant activity of benzodiazepines (but not their sedative effects) are mediated through the glycine receptor, where the benzodiazepines act as glycine agonists. However, these correlation coefficients, although statistically significant, are much lower than those reported in the previous examples. Also, rank correlations are not the most stringent technique for demonstrating meaningful relationships. For example, flunitrazepam, nitrazepam, oxazepam, and chlordiazepoxide have IC_{50}'s of 19, 20, 90, and 200 μM, respectively for inhibiting [^{3}H]strychnine binding. By ranking such IC_{50} values, rather than utilizing the absolute data themselves to calculate a correlation coefficient, one obliterates the fact that chlordiazepoxide has only one-half the potency of oxazepam whereas nitrazepam and flunitrazepam are basically identical, since each rank is given equal weight in the analysis. Furthermore, there is no other biochemical or electrophysiological data that suggests a major influence of benzodiazepines on glycine receptors (13). It thus appears that correlation coefficients on the order of 0.9 are to be expected when correlating quantitative *in vivo* and *in vitro* data if the major biochemical site for the biological activity of the drugs is being investigated.

C. Tricyclic Antidepressants: Importance of Chronic Drug Administration in Determining Interactions with Neurotransmitter Receptors

Although the major therapeutic effect of the tricyclic antidepressant is probably mediated by inhibition of the neuronal uptake mechanisms for norepinephrine and serotonin (thus increasing functional synaptic levels of these amines), their interactions with neurotransmitter receptors appear to determine their precise spectrum of activity and to modulate their effects. Paradoxically these drugs are also potent blockers of α-norepinephrine receptors in the central nervous system (CNS) (see below). This property would be expected to counteract their ability to increase norepinephrine synaptic activity. However, it is of interest that therapeutic antidepressant activity of these drugs appears only after 2 to 3 weeks of treatment. Chronic administration of such antidepressants to rats for 3 weeks leads initially to a block of α-receptors but is followed by a subsequent receptor supersensitivity, as demonstrated by an increase in α-receptor number (U'Prichard and Snyder, *personal communication*). Thus it is possible that only after 2 to 3 weeks when receptor supersensitivity develops can the increase in functional synaptic norepinephrine be manifested in an antidepressant response. This hypothesis is currently under investigation.

Studies such as this point out the complexity of using binding studies in an "acute" way to determine mechanisms of action of drugs that are given chronically in man. It is obvious that drug/receptor properties need to be studied after both acute and chronic administration for their complete spectrum of activities to be delineated (see also section IIIA).

III. RECEPTOR STUDIES AS A SCREEN FOR POTENTIAL SIDE EFFECTS

It must be emphasized that few drugs are absolutely specific in their interactions with any one neurotransmitter receptor and at therapeutic dose levels they may interact with many different receptors. In some cases this can lead to undesirable side effects whereas in other cases an interaction with another neurotransmitter system appears to be able to counteract unwanted side effects that result from interaction with the primary therapeutic site of action of the drug. Chronic drug treatments can also give rise to a spectrum of side effects that do not occur following acute dosage that appear to be mediated via changes in the receptors initially responsible for the therapeutic efficacy of the drug. In this section illustrative examples of how drug–receptor binding studies can provide important clues to the potential side effects of centrally active drugs will be discussed.

A. Side Effects Caused by Multitransmitter Receptor Interactions

1. Neuroleptics, Autonomic Side Effects, and Noradrenergic α-Receptor Binding

Autonomic sympatholytic effects such as orthostatic hypotension and sedation are among the untoward actions of neuroleptic drugs. These side effects have been attributed to blockade of central and peripheral adrenergic α-receptors (15,28) but direct quantitative evaluation of α-receptor blockade in the CNS by these agents has not been heretofore feasible. In the past year it has become possible to label the α-receptor for norepinephrine with a specific antagonist [^{3}H]WB–4101 (19). Classic α-antagonists inhibit binding of [^{3}H]WB–4101 at low concentrations in the nM range whereas β-antagonists are much weaker. Some neuroleptics are highly potent in competing for [^{3}H]WB–4101 binding to α-receptor sites in the rat brain (28). The most potent drug is the butyrophenone droperidol whose K_i value for inhibiting [^{3}H]WB–4101 binding is 0.7 nM. All the commonly used neuroleptics display K_i values under 50 nM, putting them in the same range of potency as the classic α-adrenergic antagonists phentolamine and phenoxybenzamine, whose K_i values are 3.6 and 4.0 nM respectively (46). Thus the neuroleptics, as a general class, are approximately equipotent in displacing labeled α-receptor and dopaminergic receptor antagonists.

Although the neuroleptics are potent inhibitors of α-receptor binding, their relative activity differs markedly from their relative influences in inhibiting [^{3}H]haloperidol binding. For instance, spiroperidol is the most potent neuroleptic in competing for dopamine receptor binding but is one of the weaker agents in inhibiting α-receptor binding. Droperidol is one-fourth as potent as spiroperidol at the dopamine receptor but 26 times more potent than spiroperidol at the α-receptor (28). However, pharmacological relevance can be assigned to the binding of neuroleptics to noradrenergic α-receptor.

As an index of α-receptor antagonism neuroleptics are often screened for their ability to antagonize the lethal effects of norepinephrine and epinephrine administered intravenously (21). The fatal α-adrenergic vasopressor activity of norepinephrine and epinephrine is blocked by α-antagonists such as the ergot alkaloids, phentolamine, and phenoxybenzamine but not by β-antagonists or other drugs. Similar to its stereoselectivity in inhibiting WB–4101 binding, butaclamol is also stereospecific in antagonizing epinephrine-induced mortality. The pharmacological relevance of WB–4101 binding sites is attested to by the high correlation between the potencies of neuroleptic drugs in competing for [^{3}H]WB–4101 binding and their potencies in blocking norepinephrine and epinephrine toxicity (28) ($r = 0.94$, $p < 0.001$, and $r = 0.88$, $p < 0.001$ respectively; animal data reviewed in ref. 22). This correlation across all neuroleptics is highly selective since there is no significant correlation between affinity for α-receptor binding sites and neuroleptic potency as measured in any dopamine receptor blocking tests such as catalepsy, amphetamine, or apomorphine antagonism. Similarly there is a poor correlation between neuroleptic affinity for [^{3}H]haloperidol-binding sites and antagonism of norepinephrine and epinephrine toxicity (Fig. 5).

As therapeutic brain levels of neuroleptics may be expected to correspond to concentrations of the drugs that are required to obtain an optimal blocking of dopamine receptors, the clinical propensity of neuroleptics to block α-receptors would then be related not to their absolute potencies as α-blockers, but to the ratio of their potencies as α-antagonists to their potencies as dopamine antagonists. Drugs with low ratios would be anticipated to elicit a substantial amount of α-adrenergic blockade at blood and brain levels of the drug required for adequate dopamine receptor blockade. In contrast, drugs with high ratios would be employed clinically at the very low dose levels required to secure dopamine receptor blockade and so, in general, would be less likely to elicit side effects associated with α-adrenergic blockade. Butyrophenones such as haloperidol and spiroperidol, and piperazine phenothiazines such as fluphenazine and trifluoperazine have a relatively low propensity to elicit hypotension and sedation and display ratios (K_i WB/K_i haloperidol) greater than 8 (Table 2). In contrast, promazine and clozapine, the neuroleptics with the greatest tendency to cause orthostatic hypotension and sedation, have ratios of less than 0.2. In general, the finding that alkylamino and piperidine phenothiazines are more sedating and hypotensive than the piperazine agents is manifested in the lower ratios (K_i WB/K_i haloperidol) of the former drugs. In general the butyrophenones tend to be relatively nonsedating and to have a low incidence of orthostatic hypotension and substantially higher ratios (28).

The ratio of potencies of neuroleptics *in vivo* in blocking norepinephrine toxicity to their potency in blocking amphetamine-induced stereotypy behavior has been used as a measure of their relative propensity to cause autonomic sympatho-

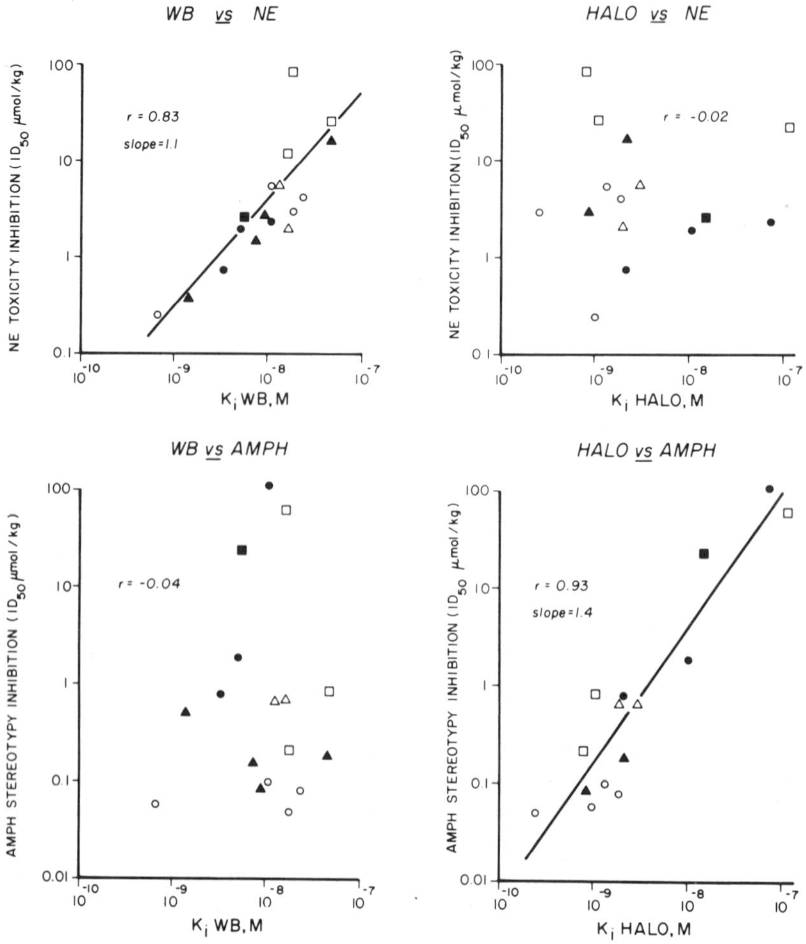

FIG. 5. Neuroleptic drugs: correlations between affinities for [^{3}H]WB-4101 rat brain binding sites and [^{3}H]haloperidol calf corpus striatum binding sites, and antagonism of norepinephrine toxicity (NE) and amphetamine stereotypy (AMPH) in the rat. [^{3}H]Haloperidol binding data and animal test data were obtained from Burt et al. (1976) and Janssen et al. (1975) respectively. The correlation coefficients $r = 0.83$ and $r = 0.93$ are significant at $p < 0.001$. Neuroleptic drug classes: phenothiazines: (●) Alkylamino. (■) Piperidine. (▲) Piperazine. (○) Butyrophenones. (△) Thioxanthenes. (□) Other.

lytic side effects (21,22). The ratio of drug potencies in these *in vivo* tests correlates highly ($r = 0.90$, $p < 0.001$) with the ratios of drug potencies in competing *in vitro* for [^{3}H]WB–4101 and [^{3}H]haloperidol binding. The slope of the correlation line is approximately 1.0, suggesting again that differential pharmacokinetic properties play a negligible role in determining the relative potencies of neuroleptics at their molecular sites of action after *in vivo* administration (28).

TABLE 2. *Relative incidence of neuroleptic-induced side effects and relative α-receptor and dopamine receptor affinity*

Drug	Sedation	Hypotension	K_iWB/K_iHalo
Dibenzodiazepines			
Clozapine	+++	+++	0.14
Phenothiazines			
Piperidine derivatives			
Thioridazine	+++	++	0.4
Alkylamino derivatives			
Chlorpromazine	+++	++	0.5
Triflupromazine	++	++	1.6
Piperazine derivatives			
Fluphenazine	+	+	11
Trifluoperazine	+	+	22
Thioxanthenes			
cis-Thiothixene	+ to ++	++	4.4
Butyrophenones			
Haloperidol	+	+	8.4
Spiroperidol	+	+	73

Adapted from ref. 28.
The highest incidence of a side effect is indicated by +++, the lowest by +.

2. *Tricyclic Antidepressants*

a. Muscarinic–Cholinergic Receptor Interactions

Tricyclic antidepressants cause considerable peripheral parasympatholytic side effects such as urinary retention, dryness of mouth, and exacerbation of glaucoma symptoms. These side effects appear to result directly from the ability of tricyclic antidepressants to block muscarinic cholinergic receptors (42). Their affinities are similar in the brain and periphery with IC_{50} concentrations ranging from 10 nM for amitriptyline to approximately 100-200 nM for desimipramine and doxepin (Table 3). The structure–activity relationships that determine anticholinergic potency are quite different from those that determine potency in inhibiting catecholamine uptake. For instance, while dimethylated drugs are more potent anticholinergics than monomethylated forms, the reverse is true for inhibition of catecholamine uptake. In contrast, dimethylated antidepressants are more potent inhibitors of serotonin uptake than are monomethylated agents. These data suggest that a drug such as amitriptyline, because of its high anticholinergic activity, would not be the antidepressant of choice for patients who also have orthostatic hypotension or glaucoma, but does support its preferential use in childhood enuresis.

There is no strong evidence that anticholinergic activity in the CNS modulates the antidepressant actions of these drugs. For example, benactyzine, an anticholinergic drug with four times greater affinity than amitriptyline for muscarinic binding sites, has minor antidepressant properties only when used in conjunction

TABLE 3. *Tricyclic antidepressants: affinity for α-noradrenergic receptors and muscarinic cholinergic receptors*

Drug	α-Receptor affinity[a]	Ability to cause psychomotor activation[b]	Sedative and hypotensive properties[b]	Muscarinic cholinergic receptor affinity[c] (nM)	
				Peripheral	Central
Tertiary amines					
Doxepin	23	—	++	100	44
Amitriptyline	24	—	++	27	10
Chlorimipramine	55	—	+	nt[d]	nt
Imipramine	58	+	+	74	78
Secondary amines					
Nortriptyline	71	++	+	100	57
Desimipramine	148	+++	—	140	170
Protriptyline	277	+++	—	nt	nt

[a] K_i inhibition [^{3}H]WB-4101 binding to rat brain (48).
[b] Detailed in ref. 47.
[c] IC_{50} inhibition [^{3}H]QNB binding to guinea pig ileum or rat brain (42).
[d] nt = not tested.

with meprobamate. However, these data point out the utility of screening potential antidepressants for muscarinic receptor binding. With all other properties being equal, a drug with low muscarinic cholinergic affinity would be clinically preferable.

b. *Noradrenergic α-Receptor Interactions*

Of the tricyclic antidepressants, the tertiary amines are particularly effective in patients with psychomotor agitation and also elicit the highest incidence of sedative and hypotensive side effects. However, the secondary amines are more effective in retarded depression since they can produce psychomotor agitation and are less likely to elicit the sedative and hypotensive side effects. Since the tertiary amine tricyclics are more potent inhibitors of serotonin uptake than the secondary amines (whereas the reverse is true for inhibition of norepinephrine uptake), it has been suggested that psychomotor activation by tricyclic antidepressants may result from blockade of norepinephrine uptake whereas the reduction of agitation is attributable to inhibition of serotonin uptake.

As already discussed, the sedative-hypotensive actions of neuroleptics appear to be related to their ability to bind to α-receptors (28). The tricyclic antidepressants are almost as potent as the neuroleptics in inhibiting the binding of [^{3}H]WB–4101 to α-noradrenergic receptors (48). Doxepin and amitriptyline (tertiary amines) are the most potent drugs with K_i values of approximately 25 nM. Protriptyline (a secondary amine), on the other hand, has a low affinity ($K_i = 280$ nM) for α-receptors. Although these data are suggestive, it is difficult to distinguish rigorously between the relative activities of these drugs in causing particular clinical effects. However, some quantitative evaluations have been performed. For example, amitriptyline is approximately three times more potent than imipramine ($K_i = 58$ nM) at α-noradrenergic receptors and relative to imipramine is approximately three times more successful in treating depression with psychomotor agitation than retarded depressions. Among six tricyclic antidepressants there is a reasonable correlation between the relative therapeutic efficacies of these drugs in relief of depression with psychomotor agitation compared to relief of depression with psychomotor inhibition and their affinities for α-noradrenergic receptors (48) (Table 3).

These data may indicate that for a given norepinephrine/serotonin uptake inhibitor a high α-adrenergic affinity would indicate a greater propensity to produce hypotensive and sedative side effects and a probable utility in treating depression associated with psychomotor agitation. Conversely, drugs with low affinity for α-noradrenergic binding sites would be predicted to have lower sedative and hypotensive properties and, lacking this braking effect, may induce only psychomotor activation and thus be more useful in treating retarded depression.

B. Side Effects Blocked by Multitransmitter Receptor Interactions: Neuroleptics, Extrapyramidal Side Effects, and Muscarinic–Cholinergic Receptor Binding

One of the most recurrent side effects of neuroleptic therapy is the Parkinsonian-like extrapyramidal side effects of rigidity and akinesia. In fact this side effect is so common that it was generally supposed that antipsychotic activity and extrapyramidal side effects were inexorably linked (39). Recently two drugs, clozapine and thioridazine, have attracted a good deal of clinical and biochemical attention. These antipsychotic agents have a much lower incidence of extrapyramidal side effects than is associated with other neuroleptic therapy. The fact that one can obtain effective antischizophrenic activity without extrapyramidal side effects led to the hypothesis that the extrapyramidal side effects and the antipsychotic activity might be mediated by dopamine receptors with slightly differing drug specificities in different regions of the brain.

Since the striatum is part of the extrapyramidal motor system it is thought the Parkinsonian side effects are probably linked with dopamine receptor blockade in the striatum. The mesolimbic areas of the forebrain (nucleus accumbens, olfactory tubercle, amygdala, and cerebral cortex) are associated classically with emotional behavior and thus these areas appear to be likely candidates for the antipsychotic activity of neuroleptics. However, studies to date (both radioreceptor and biochemical) have been conflicting and not provided much evidence to support this hypothesis. The fact that the relative affinities of clozapine and thioridazine for [^{3}H]haloperidol-binding sites in calf striatum in relation to other neuroleptics correspond reasonably well with their clinical potency indicates that these drugs probably exert their antischizophrenic effects by a mechanism similar to the other antipsychotic agents and that dopamine receptors do not differ appreciably between different brain regions. However, detailed studies with the new ligand [^{3}H]spiroperidol should be able to settle this question conclusively.

If, then, clozapine and thioridazine produce their antipsychotic effects by the same mechanisms as other neuroleptic agents, why is it that when given in therapeutic antischizophrenic doses these drugs do not produce the same incidence of extrapyramidal side effects? Recent studies of the muscarinic acetylcholine receptor in the brain may provide a resolution of this dilemma (25,41,49). It is well known that concurrent administration of anticholinergic drugs is especially effective in antagonizing the extrapyramidal side effects of neuroleptics without apparently reducing their antipsychotic potency (39). The therapeutic efficacy of the anticholinergics apparently reflects a balance in the corpus striatum between dopamine and acetylcholine involved in motor control such that antagonizing acetylcholine effects is equivalent to enhancing those of dopamine, and vice versa. Thus if neuroleptics varied in their anticholinergic properties they may well vary in their propensities to induce extrapyramidal side effects.

In studies of the binding of 3-quinuclidinyl benzilate (QNB), a potent antagonist of muscarinic cholinergic receptors, to striatal membrane preparations, this

TABLE 4. *Relative affinities of phenothiazines and butyrophenones for muscarinic cholinergic receptor binding in brain correlates inversely with extrapyramidal side effects*

Drug class	IC_{50} concentration (nM)	Frequency of extrapyramidal side effects[a]
Dibenzodiazepine		
Clozapine	26	+
Piperidine phenothiazine		
Thioridazine	150	++
Alkylamino phenothiazine		
Promazine	650	+++
Chlorpromazine	1,000	
Triflupromazine	1,000	
Piperazine phenothiazine		
Acetophenazine	10,000	++++
Perphenazine	11,000	
Trifluoperazine	13,000	
Fluphenazine	12,000	+++++
Butyrophenone		
Haloperidol	48,000	

Adapted from ref. 41.
+ = least side effects

hypothesis was confirmed. Clozapine, which is almost devoid of extrapyramidal side effects, has the greatest affinity for muscarinic receptors, quite close to that of classic anticholinergic agents (Table 4). Thioridazine, which next to clozapine elicits the fewest extrapyramidal symptoms is second most potent. The alkylamino phenothiazines, whose moderate incidence of extrapyramidal actions is greater than that of thioridazine, have correspondingly less affinity for the acetylcholine receptor. Piperazine phenothiazines and the butyrophenones, whose frequency of extrapyramidal effects is greatest, have the least affinity for the muscarinic receptors (41,49). According to this hypothesis, when given at therapeutic antischizophrenic doses all neuroleptics produce comparable dopamine receptor blockade and thus all do have about the same tendency to elicit extrapyramidal side effects. The simultaneous blockade of acetylcholine receptors by drugs such as clozapine and thioridazine antagonizes these extrapyramidal side effects, while, because of their negligible anticholinergic activity at normal doses, drugs such as haloperidol elicit many more extrapyramidal side effects. Screening of potentially useful antipsychotic drugs for muscarinic receptor affinity may thus provide a simple *in vitro* predictor of their propensity to induce extrapyramidal side effects.

C. Side Effects Caused by Chronic Influences of Drugs on Neurotransmitter Receptors: Tardive Dyskinesia and Dopamine Receptor Supersensitivity

Tardive dyskinesia is a major complication of long-term treatment with neuroleptic drugs (24). It is characterized by abnormal movements of facial muscles, tongue, and extremities that frequently worsen when the neuroleptic dose is lowered or terminated. Increasing the dose, however, may temporarily alleviate the symptoms. As an animal model of tardive dyskinesia, the chronic treatment of rats and mice with neuroleptics leads to an increased motor activity and enhanced sensitivity to the motor stimulant effect of apomorphine, a direct dopamine receptor agonist (44). A similar motor supersensitivity to dopamine receptor stimulants is apparent when dopamine synaptic activity is reduced by inhibiting synthesis of dopamine (27) or by depleting dopamine storage sites with reserpine (45). Since lesioning the nigrostriatal dopamine pathway also produces an enhanced sensitivity to dopamine receptor agonists that is hypothesized to result from a dopamine receptor supersensitivity, speculations have linked the development of tardive dyskinesia to supersensitivity of dopamine receptors after prolonged blockade by chronic drug administration (23).

In order to investigate this hypothesis directly, rats were treated for 3 weeks with the potent butyrophenone neuroleptic haloperidol (0.5 mg/kg/day). Five days after terminating the chronic treatment there was a highly significant ($p<0.001$) 20% increase in specific haloperidol binding (3). Fluphenazine, one of the most potent phenothiazine neuroleptics, produced a similar increase in binding after administration at the same dose level for 3 weeks. In contrast, treatment for 3 weeks with a fivefold higher dose of the phenothiazine promethazine, which lacks antischizophrenic activity, failed to significantly enhance [^{3}H]haloperidol binding. Depletion of brain dopamine by chronic administration of reserpine (0.2 mg/kg/day) also produced a similar 20% augmentation of [^{3}H]haloperidol binding. The enhanced receptor binding could be a reflection of either an increased number of binding sites or changes in their affinity. Scatchard analysis of saturation data indicates that it is the result of a 20 to 25% increase in the total number of binding sites with no change in affinity.

These data indicate that the motor changes seen after chronic neuroleptic treatment are associated with an increase in the number of dopamine receptor sites. This increase in the number of [^{3}H]haloperidol-binding sites is consistent with the behavioral supersensitivity to apomorphine in rats treated with a similar dose schedule of neuroleptics. However, the greater relative enhancement of apomorphine's stimulant effects in such rats compared to the increased dopamine receptor binding described here indicates that other components in the overall system determining the behavioral response may also be changed during chronic neuroleptic treatment, producing additive effects. Behavioral supersensitivity to apomorphine is more pronounced after lesions of the nigrostriatal dopamine pathway than after chronic treatment with neuroleptic drugs. Consonant with this, it has been found that following a unilateral 6-hydroxydopamine-induced lesion of the dopamine cell bodies in the substantia nigra there is a 20 to 120% increase in striatal [^{3}H]haloperidol binding 2 to 7 months following the lesion (7). This increased [^{3}H]haloperidol binding is also the result of an increased number of binding sites. Rats that are more behaviorally supersensitive also tend to show a greater increase in dopamine receptor binding.

Thus it is possible that enhanced dopamine receptor binding following chronic drug treatment may be a useful *in vitro* predictor of *in vivo* propensity to produce tardive dyskinesia.

In conducting chronic drug studies it is important to ensure that the animals are healthy at the time of assay so that any biochemical changes are not the result of nonspecific effects such as dehydration or malnutrition. In studies where receptor antagonists have been utilized it is important that, at the point of assay, remaining drug in the brain is removed, either by a drug-free period *in vivo* or by centrifugation washes of brain membranes *in vitro.* In the previous example if haloperidol had not been removed by such procedures, then the increase in receptors would have been masked by the haloperidol binding to these sites at the time of assay. If possible, brain or membrane levels of drug used in the chronic treatment period should be measured directly in the final tissue preparation. Drug dosage in the chronic treatment period should also correspond approximately to human dose levels or to levels that produce behavioral effects that have previously been used in the animals as *in vivo* screens for therapeutic activity.

VI. DIFFERENTIATION OF AGONISTS FROM ANTAGONISTS USING RECEPTOR-BINDING ASSAYS

In classic receptor theory, binding studies of a simple receptor give information only of a drug's affinity for its binding site. There is no measure of its intrinsic activity. In other words, two drugs may exhibit the same affinity for a receptor but one may be an agonist and the other an antagonist—an important pharmacological distinction! However, it has proved possible to use receptor-binding assays to distinguish agonists from antagonists and many of the neurotransmitter receptors that have been studied do not appear to be "classically simple."

A. Opiates: "The Sodium Shift"

Unlike the neuroleptics that bear little resemblence to the agonist dopamine, opiate agonists and antagonists are very similar chemically. For instance, the addition of an allyl group to the *N*-methyl of the potent opiate agonist oxymorphone produces naloxone, a pure opiate antagonist with no analgesic activity. Not surprisingly, early studies of opiate binding to brain membranes found that pharmacologically potent opiates, whether agonists or antagonists, bound with similar high affinity to apparently identical receptors (30,36). These initial studies were conducted in a sodium-free medium. However, when physiological concentrations of sodium were added, opiate agonists became weaker whereas opiate antagonist affinity remained constant (29). This suggested an *in vitro* method to distinguish opiate agonists from antagonists.

The influence of sodium on unlabeled opiate binding can be investigated by determining the potency of the drug in inhibiting the binding of [^{3}H]naloxone to opiate receptors in the presence and the absence of sodium (31). Opiate agonists become between 9 to 60 times weaker at inhibiting [^{3}H]naloxone binding in the presence of sodium, whereas the potency of pure antagonists remains unchanged (or increases slightly, in some cases) (Table 5). Opiates are interesting in that a number of compounds demonstrate both agonist and antagonist properties. For example nalorphine (morphine with the exchange of an *N*-allyl group for the *N*-methyl) is an agonist in its own right and at high doses can cause analgesia but, at low doses, it can also block morphine analgesia and cause withdrawal in opiate addicts. Opiate antagonists with more agonist activity than nalorphine such as pentozocine (sodium shift = 3.3) appear to be more clinically useful than pure opiate agonists, such as morphine, as they have a lower tendency to cause addiction. Animal screens for analgesic activity of such mixed agonist–antagonists have proven somewhat complicated, since their analgetic activity is sometimes only demonstrable under very precise conditions (such as a particular temperature in the hot-plate test) or not at all in some test situations, where morphine is active. These drugs are clearly differentiated in opiate-binding assays as their potency in inhibiting [^{3}H]naloxone binding is reduced between three- and sevenfold by the addition of 100 mM NaCl. In general "sodium shifts" of

TABLE 5. *Effects of sodium ion on inhibition by opiate agonists and antagonists of stereospecific [^{3}H]naloxone binding to rat brain homogenates*

Nonradioactive opiate	IC_{50} of stereospecific [^{3}H]naloxone binding (nM): No NaCl	100 mM NaCl	Sodium shift IC_{50} ratio, +NaCl/−NaCl
Pure antagonists			
Naloxone	1.5	1.5	1.0
Naltrexone	0.5	0.5	1.0
Diprenorphine	0.5	0.5	1.0
Mixed agonists–antagonists			
Cyclazocine	0.9	1.5	1.7
Levallorphan	1.0	2.0	2.0
Nalorphine	1.5	4.0	2.7
Pentazocine	15	50	3.3
Metazocine	10	60	6.0
Pure agonists			
Met-enkephalin	50	450	9
Etorphine	0.5	6.0	12
Phenazocine	0.6	8.0	13
Meperidine	3,000	50,000	17
Leu-enkephalin	12.0	225	19
D-Ala^2-enkephalin	5.3	140	26
Methadone	7.0	200	28
Morphine	3.0	110	37
(±)-Propoxyphene	200	12,000	60

Experimental data are modified and updated from ref. 31.

between one and two characterize opiate antagonists with very little or no agonist activity.

This simple "sodium index" provides a straightforward *in vitro* means of predicting the extent to which an opiate may be an agonist or antagonist. As yet it is unclear what the significance of differences in sodium shifts indicates among pure agonists. For example, etorphine has a sodium shift of 12 and morphine a shift of 37, yet both appear to be pure agonists. It is important to point out that these sodium shifts, and for that matter, any drug affinity for a particular receptor, are determined under certain, precise conditions. Any deviation from these conditions will change the absolute values of these quantities although, in general, the results will be qualitatively similar (10,34).

The discovery of the opiate peptides, enkephalins and endorphins, has opened the possibility that there may also be other states of the opiate receptor to which these peptides bind, or, in fact, other opiate receptors of differing specificities. Indeed, the pituitary opiate receptors have a lower affinity for morphine and the enkephalins than do brain opiate receptors although β-endorphin has the same affinity in both regions (35). In labeling brain opiate receptors with [^{3}H]enkephalins differences among opiate agonists are evident. For example, whereas etorphine is equipotent at displacing [^{3}H]dihydromorphine and [^{3}H]met-enkephalin binding, morphine is much weaker at displacing [^{3}H]met-enkephalin binding than [^{3}H]dihydromorphine binding. Thus in screens for synthetic opioid peptide activity [^{3}H]enkephalin binding must also be investigated.

These data clearly indicate that binding studies can differentiate among opiate antagonists and agonists in a number of ways. The significance of these results in regard to the mechanism of opiate/enkephalin/endorphin action are not yet clear (38). However, opiate receptor-binding assays can clearly distinguish drugs that will have opiate activity *in vivo* from drugs that will not. The sodium shift is often suggestive of the particular spectrum of pharmacological effects the drug will exhibit and may pick out those drugs that will have a lower potential for addiction for further animal studies.

B. Differential Affinity of Agonist Versus Antagonist Ligands

As we have just seen, opiate agonists can be distinguished from antagonists by the differential influence of sodium. These data clearly indicate that the opiate receptor is not a simple classic single-binding site but that the receptor either interconverts or possibly exists in two distinct forms with differential agonist or antagonist affinities (see Chapter 2).

This may also be a feature of other neurotransmitter receptors (37). For example, in labeling the dopamine receptor with the antagonist [^{3}H]haloperidol, agonists, as a group, have low affinity (2,4) for these binding sites, whereas antagonists, as a group, have high affinity. The reverse holds true if the receptor is labeled with the agonist [^{3}H]dopamine. Then agonists, as a group, demonstrate high affinity and antagonists low affinity (2,4). This reciprocity of relative affinity appears to hold true for the α-norepinephrine receptor, the muscarinic–cholinergic receptor, and the serotonin receptor.

Such findings immediately suggest that, for example, a specific and potent dopamine agonist, which would have utility as an antiparkinson drug, could be screened for by selecting an agent with high affinity for [^{3}H]dopamine-binding sites. Unfortunately this does not appear to be correct. Bromokryptine is a potent dopamine agonist *in vivo* yet it has a relatively lower affinity for [^{3}H]dopamine-binding sites than for [^{3}H]haloperidol-binding sites (2). According to the previous hypothesis this result would be predictive of antagonist, or at best, mixed agonist–antagonist activity. However, recent data are suggesting that the high-affinity agonist-binding sites for both the dopamine and the α-noradrenergic receptors may represent desensitized and nonpharmacologically relevant receptors (8). Thus the high affinity of bromokryptine for [^{3}H]haloperidol-binding sites should be interpreted as indicative of potent dopaminergic activity, but the question of its agonist or antagonist profile can only be answered by *in vivo* animal tests.

However, bromokryptine is only one drug, and its complex interactions with other neurotransmitter receptors such as the serotonin and noradrenergic receptors (47), as well as its effects on amine release, may be a complicating factor. Studies of agonist/antagonist-binding sites are still at a developmental stage and may yet prove to be of utility in the search for novel therapeutic agents.

V. CONCLUSION AND CAVEAT

As we have seen, for drugs that exert their effects by interacting directly with neurotransmitter receptors, binding assays provide an inexpensive, rapid, and efficient *in vitro* screening procedure. Detailed structure–activity analyses, unencumbered by problems of absorption and metabolism, can quickly focus on the active centers of a drug that may be amenable to further chemical refinement. It could be argued that such binding studies will provide only more of the same types of drugs that are already available. This is true, in part, but, for example, opiate receptor-binding studies have already spurred on the development of the novel peptide opiates. The same stimulation may be exerted in the development of "benzodiazepine–receptor ligand" analogs. Furthermore there are receptors for such putative neurotransmitters as angiotensin, neurotensin, or TRH which have already been characterized that remain in search of both specific drugs and diseases. Also, "seminovel" compounds are needed that embody the characteristics that have been determined to be responsible for their therapeutic utility (e.g., dopamine receptor blocking activity for neuroleptics) but that have differing affinities for other neurotransmitter receptors. For example, the ideal neuroleptic might probably have high dopamine receptor affinity and high cholinergic receptor activity but low α-norepinephrine receptor affinity, and not result in dopamine receptor supersensitivity following chronic treatments.

Of course, receptor-binding assays cannot replace *in vivo* testing. A potent drug discovered *in vitro* may not be absorbed or cross the blood–brain barrier, or may be rapidly metabolized *in vivo.* On the other hand a precursor, such as L-DOPA, which may be metabolized *in vivo* to an active agent would be missed by *in vitro* screens. It would be unlikely that an aphrodisiac would be discovered while conducting a receptor-binding study, although an astute observer may notice such activity while performing many *in vivo* screens. Receptor-binding techniques are probably best thought of as methods by which to understand the therapeutic mechanism of some drugs and that may then aid in their refinement. As such, they have surely earned a place as a very useful tool in the laboratories of psychopharmacologists and the pharmaceutical industry.

VI. SUMMARY

Behavioral, electrophysiological, and pharmacological studies have indicated that many psychoactive drugs produce their effects by interacting with (neurotransmitter) receptors in the brain. The absolute potencies of a series of drugs *in vivo* can be compared to the profile of absolute drug affinities at a drug or neurotransmitter receptor-binding site. A high correlation between such *in vivo* and *in vitro* data is suggestive that such a binding site is the biochemical locus for the *in vivo* activity of the drug series. As such, affinity for this binding site can be used as a screen for novel compounds that may show similar *in vivo* activity. Such drug receptor screens allow detailed structure–activity relationships to be determined *in vitro* without the problems of metabolism and absorption that complicate *in vivo* studies. Such studies allow the pinpointing of the active sites within the drug molecule for further synthetic manipulations. Receptor-binding screens are rapid, inexpensive, and only milligram quantities of novel compounds need to be synthesized for study.

Receptor-binding screens for the biochemical locus responsible for therapeutic drug action have demonstrated that neuroleptic affinity for brain dopamine receptors correlates highly with *in vivo* antipsychotic activity in schizophrenics. Benzodiazepines, however, have specific binding sites, affinity for which correlates with *in vivo* activity but which have yet to be related to a specific neurotransmitter. Drug side effects can also be related to neurotransmitter receptor interaction and thus binding studies can screen for this potential. Neuroleptic interactions with α-adrenergic receptors is predictive of sympatholytic side effects, whereas chronic neuroleptic treatment can lead to increases in dopamine receptor number that may be responsible for tardive dyskinesia. Multitransmitter receptor interactions can be beneficial, in some cases, since high affinity of neuroleptic drugs for muscarinic–cholinergic receptors decreases their extrapyramidal side effects. The precise clinical profile of tricyclic antidepressants is also modulated by various neurotransmitter receptor interactions. Receptor-binding screens can also be used to distinguish agonists from antagonists, as in the case of the "sodium shift" that distinguishes opiate analgesics from their antagonists.

Receptor-binding screens have much potential for determining the biochemical locus for the therapeutic effects of many psychoactive drugs. As such they will provide excellent *in vitro* screens to enable the pharmaceutical industry to develop new, potent, and specific drugs with fewer side effects.

VII. REFERENCES

1. Bennett, J. P., Jr., and Snyder, S. H. (1975): Stereospecific binding of d-lysergic acid diethylamide (LSD) to brain membranes: Relationship to serotonin receptors. *Brain Res.,* 94:523–544.
2. Burt, D. R., Creese, I., and Snyder, S. (1976): Characteristics of ^{3}H-haloperidol and ^{3}H-dopamine binding associated with dopamine receptors in calf brain membranes. *Mol. Pharmacol.,* 12:800–812.
3. Burt, D. R., Creese, I., and Snyder, S. H. (1977): Antischizophrenic drugs: Chronic treatment elevates dopamine receptor binding in brain. *Science,* 196:326–328.
4. Creese, I., Burt, D. R., and Snyder, S. H. (1975): Dopamine receptor binding: Differentiation of agonist and antagonist states with ^{3}H-dopamine and ^{3}H-haloperidol. *Life Sci.,* 17:993–1002.
5. Creese, I., Burt, D. R., and Snyder, S. H. (1976): Dopamine receptor binding predicts clinical and pharmacological potencies of antischizophrenic drugs. *Science,* 192:481–483.
6. Creese, I., Burt, D. R., and Snyder, S. H. (1976): Dopamine receptors and average clinical doses. *Science,* 194:546.
7. Creese, I., Burt, D. R., and Snyder, S. H. (1977): Dopamine receptor binding enhancement accompanies lesion-induced behavioral supersensitivity. *Science,* 197:596–598.
8. Creese, I., Burt, D. R., and Snyder, S. H. (1978): Biochemical actions of neuroleptic drugs: focus on the dopamine receptor. In: *Handbook of Psychopharmacology,* Vol. 10, edited by L. L. Iversen, S. D. Iversen, and S. H. Snyder, pp. 37–89. Plenum Press, New York.
9. Creese, I., Feinberg, A., and Snyder, S. H. (1976): Butyrophenone influences on the opiate receptor. *Eur. J. Pharmacol.,* 36:231–235.
10. Creese, I., Pasternak, G. W., Pert, C. B., and Snyder, S. H. (1975): Discrimination by temperature of opiate agonist and antagonist receptor binding. *Life Sci.,* 16:1837–1842.
11. Creese, I., Schneider, R., and Snyder, S. H. (1977): ^{3}H-Spiroperidol labels dopamine receptors in pituitary and brain. *Eur. J. Pharmacol.,* 46:377–381.
12. Creese, I., and Snyder, S. H. (1977): A novel, simple and sensitive radioreceptor assay for antischizophrenic drugs in blood. *Nature (Lond),* 270:180–182.
13. Curtis, D. R., Game, C. J. A., and Lodge, D. (1976): Benzodiazepines and central glycine receptors. *Br. J. Pharmacol.,* 56:307–311.
14. Deniker, P. (1970): Introduction of neuroleptic chemotherapy into psychiatry. In: *Discoveries in Biological Psychiatry,* edited by F. J. Ayd, Jr. and B. Blackwell, pp. 155–164, Lippincott, Philadelphia.
15. Ebert, M. H., and Shader, R. I. (1970): Cardiovascular effects. In: *Psychotropic Drug Side Effects,* edited by R. I. Shader and A. DiMascio, pp. 149–163. Williams & Wilkins, Baltimore.
16. Enna, S. J., Bennett, J. P., Jr., Burt, D. R., Creese, I., and Snyder, S. H. (1976): Stereospecificity of interaction of neuroleptic drugs with neurotransmitters and correlation with clinical potency. *Nature (Lond),* 263:338–341.
17. Enna, S. J., Creese, I., U'Prichard, D. C., Greenberg, D. A., and Snyder, S. H. (1977): Stereospecificity and clinical potency of neuroleptics—a reply. *Nature (Lond),* 267:183–184.
18. Fields, J. Z., Reisine, T. D., and Yamamura, H. I. (1977): Biochemical demonstration of dopaminergic receptors in rat and human brain using ^{3}H-spiroperidol. *Brain Res.,* 136:578–584.
19. Greenberg, D. A., U'Prichard, D. C., and Snyder, S. H. (1976): α-Noradrenergic receptor binding in mammalian brain, differential labeling of agonist and antagonist states. *Life Sci.,* 19:69–76.
20. Janssen, P. A. J. (1970): The butyrophenone story. In: *Discoveries in Biological Psychiatry,* edited by F. J. Ayd and B. Blackwell, pp. 165–176. Lippincott, Philadelphia.

21. Janssen, P. A. J., Neimegeers, C. J. E., and Schellekens, K. H. L. (1965): Is it possible to predict the clinical effects of neuroleptic drugs (major tranquilizers) from animal action? Part 1. *Arzneim. Forsch.*, 15:104–117.
22. Janssen, P. A. J., and Van Bever, N. F. (1975): Advances in the search for improved neuroleptic drugs. In: *Current Developments in Psychopharmacology*, Vol. 2, edited by W. B. Essman and L. Valzelli, pp. 165 184. Spectrum, New York.
23. Klawans, H. L. (1973): The pharmacology of tardive dyskinesias. *Am. J. Psychiatry*, 130:82–86.
24. Kobayashi, R. K. (1977): Drug therapy of tardive dyskinesia. *N. Engl. J. Med.*, 296:257–260.
25. Miller, R. J., and Hiley, C. R. (1974): Anti-muscarinic properties of neuroleptics and drug-induced parkinsonism. *Nature (Lond)*, 248:596–597.
26. Mohler, H., and Okada, T. (1977): Benzodiazepine receptor in the central nervous system. *Science*, 198:849–851.
27. Moore, K. E., and Thornburg, J. E. (1975): Drug induced dopaminergic supersensitivity. In: *Advances in Neurology Vol. 9*, edited by D. Calne, T. N. Chase, and A. Barbeau, pp. 93–104. Raven press, New York.
28. Peroutka, S. J., U'Prichard, D. C., Greenberg, D. A., and Snyder, S. H. (1977): Neuroleptic drug interactions with norepinephrine α-receptor binding sites in rat brain. *Neuropharmacology*, 16:549–556.
29. Pert, C. B., Pasternak, G. W., and Snyder, S. H. (1973): Opiate agonists and antagonists discriminated by receptor binding in brain. *Science*, 182:1359–1361.
30. Pert, C. B., and Snyder, S. H. (1973): Opiate receptor: Demonstration in nervous tissue. *Science*, 179:1011–1014.
31. Pert, C. B., and Snyder, S. H. (1974): Opiate receptor binding of agonists and antagonists affected differentially by sodium. *Mol. Pharmacol.*, 10:868–879.
32. Seeman, P., Chau-Wong, M., Tedesco, J., and Wong, K. (1975): Brain receptors for antipsychotic drugs and dopamine: Direct binding assays. *Proc. Natl. Acad. Sci. USA*, 72:4376–4380.
33. Seeman, P., Lee, T., Chau-Wong, M., and Wong, K. (1976): Antipsychotic drug doses and neuroleptic/dopamine receptors. *Nature (Lond)*, 261:717–719.
34. Simantov, R., Snowman, A. M., and Snyder, S. H. (1976): Temperature and ionic influences on opiate receptor binding. *Mol. Pharmacol.*, 12:977–986.
35. Simantov, R., and Snyder, S. H. (1977): Opiate receptor binding in the pituitary gland. *Brain Res.*, 124:178–184.
36. Simon, E., Hiller, J., and Edelman, I. (1973): Stereospecific binding of the potent narcotic analgesic ^{3}H-etorphine to rat brain homogenates. *Proc. Natl. Acad. Sci. USA*, 70:1947–1949.
37. Snyder, S. H. (1975): Neurotransmitter and drug receptors in the brain. *Biochem. Pharmacol.*, 24:1371–1374.
38. Snyder, S. H. (1977): Opiate receptors in the brain. *N. Engl. J. Med.*, 296:266–271.
39. Snyder, S. H., Banerjee, S. P., Yamamura, H. I., and Greenberg, D. (1974): Drugs, neurotransmitters and schizophrenia. *Science*, 184:1243–1253.
40. Snyder, S. H., Creese, I., and Burt, D. R. (1975): The brain's dopamine receptor: Labeling with ^{3}H-dopamine and ^{3}H-haloperidol. *Psychopharmacol. Commun.*, 1:663–673.
41. Snyder, S. H., Greenberg, D., and Yamamura, H. I. (1976): Antischizophrenic drugs and brain cholinergic receptors. *Arch. Gen. Psychiatry*, 31:58–61.
42. Snyder, S. H., and Yamamura, H. I. (1977): Antidepressants and the muscarinic acetylcholine receptor. *Arch. Gen. Psychiatry*, 34:236–239.
43. Squires, R., and Braestrup, C. (1977): Benzodiazepine receptor in rat brain. *Nature (Lond)*, 266:732–734.
44. Tarsey, D., and Baldessarini, R. J. (1974): Behavioral supersensitivity to apomorphine following chronic treatment with drugs which interfere with the synaptic function of catecholamines. *Neuropharmacology*, 13:927–940.
45. Ungerstedt, U., Ljungberg, T., Hoffer, B., and Siggins, G. (1975): Dopamine supersensitivity in the striatum. *Adv. Neurol.*, 9:57–66.
46. U'Prichard, D. C., Greenberg, D. A., and Snyder, S. H. (1977): Binding characteristics of a radiolabeled agonist and antagonist at central nervous system alpha noradrenergic receptors. *Mol. Pharmacol.*, 13:454–473.
47. U'Prichard, D. C., and Snyder, S. H. (1977): Therapeutic and side effects of psychotropic drugs: the relevance of receptor binding methodology. In: *Animal Models in Psychiatry and Neurology*, edited by I. Hamin and E. Usdin, pp. 477–495. Pergamon Press, New York.

48. U'Prichard, D. C., Greenberg, D. A., Sheenan, P. P., and Snyder, S. H. (1977): Tricyclic antidepressants: Correlation of therapeutic properties with affinity for alpha-noradrenergic receptor binding sites in the brain. *Science,* 199:197–198.
49. Yamamura, H. I., Manian, A. A., and Snyder, S. H. (1976): Muscarinic cholinergic receptor binding: Influence of pimozide and chlorpromazine metabolites. *Life Sci.,* 18:685–692.
50. Young, A. B., and Snyder, S. H. (1973): Strychnine binding associated with glycine receptors of the central nervous system. *Proc. Natl. Acad. Sci. USA,* 70:2832–2836.
51. Young, A. B., Zukin, S. R., and Snyder, S. H. (1974): Interactions of benzodiazepines with central nervous system glycine receptors: Possible mechanism of action. *Proc. Natl. Acad. Sci. USA,* 71:2246–2250.

Neurotransmitter Receptor Binding, edited by
H. I. Yamamura et al.
Raven Press, New York © 1978.

9

Other Uses of Neurotransmitter Receptor-Binding Assays

Henry I. Yamamura

Department of Pharmacology, College of Medicine, University of Arizona Health Sciences Center, Tucson, Arizona 85724

I. INTRODUCTION

As shown throughout this book, neurotransmitter receptor-binding assays have been used as tools in solving many of the problems in neurobiology and pharmacology. For example, as pointed out by Enna in Chapter 7, receptor-binding assay procedures can be used as radioreceptor assays for the detection of endogenous neurotransmitter substances. Creese has indicated in Chapter 8 that receptor-binding assays are useful as tools for determining the mechanism of action of certain drugs. For example, a specific high-affinity binding assay for the benzodiazepines has recently become available (40,48,49). Through use of this assay it may be possible to isolate an endogenous "anti-anxiety" factor that normally acts at this binding site.

Receptor-binding assays can also be useful as screening methods for determining the drug side effects. For example, the sedation and hypotension produced by various neuroleptics have been attributed to their blockade of central and peripheral α-adrenergic receptors (57). The expression of Parkinsonian-like extrapyramidal side effects of some neuroleptics has been attributed to their lack of effect at the central muscarinic cholinergic receptor (47).

The receptor-binding assays may also be used to detect neurotransmitter receptor alterations in animals after chronic drug treatment. Burt et al. (9) have chronically treated animals with a dopaminergic antagonist, haloperidol, and have reported dopamine receptor supersensitivity in selected areas of the brain, suggesting that enhanced dopamine receptor binding in the basal ganglia may be a useful *in vitro* predictor of *in vivo* propensity to produce tardive dyskinesia.

In this introductory section I have briefly cited several examples illustrated in this book in which the receptor-binding assay has been a useful tool. In this chapter, I would like to point out other examples that suggest possible directions for future work.

II. DEVELOPMENTAL STUDIES

Synaptogenesis in the mammalian central nervous system (CNS) has been an area of interest. Previous biochemical analyses during development were focused mainly on the levels of neurotransmitter substances and on the activity of their biosynthetic and degradative enzymes. The interrelationship between the presynaptic and postsynaptic elements in the ontogeny of synapses, however, is still a major question in developmental neurobiology. With the advent of highly sensitive neurotransmitter receptor-binding assays, it is now possible to examine the development of the pre- and postsynaptic components of various neurotransmitter systems. Several such studies have recently been reported (12,26,27,44).

A. Muscarinic Cholinergic Receptors in Developing Rat Brain

For developmental studies, Sprague-Dawley female rats, sperm positive on a specific date, may be purchased from a commercial source and the animals placed in separate cages after 16 days of gestation.

In characterizing specific muscarinic receptors with [^{3}H]quinuclidinyl benzilate ([^{3}H]QNB), several items of interest should be considered (65). Since [^{3}H]QNB can bind to lower affinity nonspecific sites as well as to the high-affinity muscarinic cholinergic receptors, the amount of nonspecific binding should be assessed by carrying out parallel incubations in the presence of oxotremorine (100 μM), a potent muscarinic agonist, or atropine (1.0 μM), a competitive muscarinic antagonist. Since 0.5 nM is a near-saturating concentration of [^{3}H]QNB the amount of [^{3}H]QNB specifically bound should reflect the number of available muscarinic receptors in the assay. This may not be the case, however, if a lower affinity atropine-sensitive binding site also exists in the tissue. Saturation studies and subsequent Scatchard analyses should be performed at several developmental stages to determine if there is more than one class of sites. These analyses will also indicate if any change in specific receptors during development is due to a change in the density of receptors or to a change in the affinity of [^{3}H]QNB for the muscarinic receptor. To insure specificity at the early stages of development, the stereospecificity of pharmacological agents should be examined in receptor binding. For example, this can easily be done for the cholinergic system by using dexetimide and levetimide, the pharmacological stereoisomers of benzetimide. At nanomolar concentrations, only the pharmacologically active isomer, dexetimide, should be effective in displacing [^{3}H]QNB from the muscarinic receptor whereas the pharmacologically inactive isomer, levetimide, should be ineffective at these concentrations (44).

With respect to the development of muscarinic cholinergic synapses in rat brain, the postsynaptic receptor has recently been compared to the development of three presynaptic parameters: choline acetyltransferase activity, endogenous acetylcholine levels, and the high-affinity, sodium-dependent [^{3}H]choline transport system (12). At 15 days of gestation, the brain exhibits low but detectable levels of specific [^{3}H]QNB binding. The receptor density increases in a linear fashion during the last week of gestation and the first month after birth, reaching adult levels at the same time as acetylcholine. The concentrations of muscarinic agonists and antagonists necessary to inhibit [^{3}H]QNB binding by 50% (IC_{50}) are not significantly different in the neonatal and adult brain preparations, suggesting that the muscarinic receptor-binding site is being measured throughout the developmental stages.

By comparing the pre- and postsynaptic elements during development, it may be possible to learn if one neuron influences the development of another neuron. For example, when cholinergic parameters of the synapse were examined, the development of the muscarinic receptor in whole brain paralleled but preceded the development of choline acetyltransferase activity and [^{3}H]choline uptake (12). In all brain regions examined, the receptor levels reached adult concentrations well before the activity of choline acetyltransferase did.

Extensive studies *in vivo* and *in vitro* of the neuromuscular junction indicate that the nicotinic cholinergic receptor, too, appears on the muscle membrane prior to the development of cholinergic innervation (17,23). If the activity of choline acetyltransferase is a reliable index of presynaptic cholinergic development, then the development of the postsynaptic muscarinic cholinergic receptor appears to precede innervation by the presynaptic neuron.

B. β-Adrenergic Receptors in Developing Rat Brain

Another interesting way of studying receptor development is to correlate the recognition site changes with the biochemical activity of the receptor [e.g., the formation of cyclic-3′,5′-adenosine monophosphate (cyclic AMP)]. The ontogeny of β-adrenergic receptors in the rat cerebral cortex has been studied using the β-adrenergic antagonist ^{125}I-hydroxybenzylpindolol (26). The affinities of L-isoproterenol (a β-receptor agonist) and iodohydroxybenzylpindolol for the β-adrenergic receptor did not change throughout with development of the animal. In contrast to the muscarinic cholinergic receptor, which reached adulthood levels after one month of postnatal development, the density of β-adrenergic receptors reached adult levels in the second week of postnatal development. And while norepinephrine-stimulated cyclic AMP followed closely the development of the β-adrenergic receptor, norepinephrine stores in the cerebral cortex reached adulthood only after 2 months of postnatal development. Thus the ontogenic pattern of the β-adrenergic receptor and the second messenger paralleled each other but did not correlate with the time course of development of norepinephrine stores. Further research will determine the significance of and the reason for this lack of correlation.

III. THE QUESTION OF "SPARE" NEUROTRANSMITTER RECEPTORS

An interesting question in receptor theory has to do with the existence of "spare" neurotransmitter receptors. This concept emerged from pharmacological studies using primarily the isolated guinea pig ileum preparation (24). Pharmacological evidence suggests that a drug might elicit maximal contractions of the intestine while occupying only a small percentage (5 to 10%) of the total available receptor sites, with the remainder termed "spare" receptors. The question of spare receptors may be answered by the use of neurotransmitter receptor-binding assays. To achieve this, *in vitro* binding assays are performed using a potent neurotransmitter agonist that acts on tissues (guinea pig ileum) and the findings are compared with the biological response of the agonist on the same tissue. If a low concentration of the agonist produces 10% specific binding in an *in vitro* binding assay and also produces a full biological response in the muscle, then the existence of spare receptors would be suggested. If, on the other hand, at a concentration at which 50% of the total binding sites are occupied, and the agonist elicits 50% of its maximal pharmacological effect, then the existence of spare receptors could not be supported. Another approach to this problem may include the evaluation of a biological response by an agonist before and after irreversible blockade of the receptor, at a concentration irreversibly inhibiting, say, 80% of the neurotransmitter receptors. If the agonist can still produce a maximal biological response even though at most only 20% of the receptors are occupied, then the existence of spare receptors would again be indicated. Using this procedure, spare opiate receptors have not been found in the guinea pig ileum preparation (14).

IV. EXISTENCE OF PRESYNAPTIC NEUROTRANSMITTER RECEPTORS

Neurotransmitter receptors in the CNS have traditionally been thought to be located postsynaptically on dendrites or soma of neurons that receive synaptic input from presynaptic nerve endings that contain a given neurotransmitter. Recent evidence suggests that presynaptic neurotransmitter receptors also exist and that they may function physiologically as part of a negative feedback system to modulate transmitter release (11). In some tissues in the peripheral sympathetic nervous system and in brain slices from some areas, adrenergic antagonists enhance norepinephrine release whereas adrenergic agonists including norepinephrine itself diminish release (21,31,50–52). In brain slices of the cerebral cortex, atropine enhances acetylcholine release whereas the muscarinic agonist, oxotremorine, and the acetylcholinesterase inhibitor, physostigmine, reduce acetylcholine release (38,39,41,54). There are data showing that bicuculline, the γ-aminobutyric acid (GABA) receptor antagonist, enhances the efflux of GABA from brain slices (30). All of these pharmacological observations suggest that neurotransmitters released into the synaptic cleft not only interact with the postsynaptic receptor but also may act upon receptor sites on the presynaptic neuron to prevent further transmitter release. This feedback would provide a valuable direct and immediate means of modulating transmitter release; other proposed feedback mechanisms require recurrent neuronal pathways from the postsynaptic cell back to the presynaptic cell body.

To determine by direct binding assays whether or not muscarinic cholinergic receptors are located on the presynaptic afferent neurons projecting to the hippocampus, it is convenient to study the septal–hippocampal cholinergic tract in the CNS (35,36). If afferent neurons do contain muscarinic receptors, then destruction of these fibers by electrolytic lesions of the medial septum should decrease the density of measurable muscarinic receptors in the hippocampus. Just such an attempt to demonstrate presynaptic muscarinic cholinergic receptors has been reported (66). The choline acetyltransferase activity was reduced approximately 75% in the hippocampal homogenates 2, 9, and 14 days after septal lesion, demonstrating a loss of nerve endings; specific [^{3}H]QNB binding, however, was unaltered. Several types of experiments were carried out in an effort to explain the unaltered state of the binding (66).

What are the possible explanations for the failure to detect alterations in specific [^{3}H]QNB binding in the septal lesioned hippocampus? On the one hand, the lack of any reduction in muscarinic cholinergic receptors after septal lesions, which destroyed the majority of the cholinergic input to the hippocampus, might argue against the existence of presynaptic muscarinic receptors on cholinergic neurons in the hippocampus. On the other hand, it is conceivable that presynaptic muscarinic binding sites have different binding properties than the postsynaptic receptors and that the presynaptic sites were not labeled to any appreciable extent with the low concentrations of [^{3}H]ligand used in the experiment. In this respect, Szerb and co-workers (53) have recently examined the effects of QNB on [^{3}H]acetylcholine release from hippocampal slices after preloading the tissue with [^{3}H]choline. They reported that the concentration of QNB required to inhibit [^{3}H]acetylcholine release 50% was 10 nM. In a recent study, the dissociation constant of [^{3}H]QNB for the postsynaptic muscarinic receptor has been shown to be less than 50 pM (22).

There is the further possibility that presynaptic muscarinic receptors may exist on noncholinergic neurons. This has recently been shown to be the case. Sharma and Banerjee (45) were able to demonstrate a 50% decrease in specific [^{3}H]QNB binding in the heart after destruction of the sympathetic nerve terminals with 6-hydroxydopamine. How can one show that the decreases in [^{3}H]QNB binding in the heart after 6-hydroxydopamine (6-OHDA) were not due to decreases in the density of postsynaptic muscarinic receptors caused by unaltered regulation by the noradrenergic neurons? To answer this question Sharma and Banerjee (45) pretreated animals with reserpine, which destroys the storage mechanisms for catecholamines in the sympathetic nerve terminals. Chronic reserpine treatment did not alter specific [^{3}H]QNB binding in the heart, indicating that sympathetic transmission was not involved in the regulation of the postsynaptic muscarinic receptors. Therefore, they concluded from these studies that the decrease in [^{3}H]QNB binding in the heart following chemical sympathectomy was due to the loss of presynaptic muscarinic receptors located on noradrenergic terminals. Further studies should determine the similarity between the pre- and postsynaptic receptors.

V. SIMILARITY OF CENTRAL AND PERIPHERAL NEUROTRANSMITTER RECEPTORS.

Because there is pharmacological evidence that the nicotinic cholinergic receptors in the sympathetic ganglia are different from the nicotinic receptors located on the neuromuscular junction, the question can be asked whether muscarinic receptors located in the periphery are similar to those located in the brain. For comparison of central and peripheral receptors, one should determine the dissociation constants using the several available methods as given in Chapter 4, and examine the pharmacological specificity of certain drugs and the stereospecificity of certain pharmacological isomers.

For characterizing a peripheral receptor, one can examine the muscarinic receptors in the heart. It is well known that the vagus nerve innervating the myocardium releases acetylcholine which interacts with receptors producing negative inotropic and chronotropic responses. These effects are blocked by the muscarinic antagonist atropine. Other peripheral tissues that one can also examine for muscarinic receptors are the smooth muscle, a well characterized example of which is the longitudinal muscle of the guinea pig ileum, and the exocrine glands.

Several investigators have recently examined the specific binding of muscarinic antagonists such as [^{3}H]atropine (4), [^{3}H]QNB (22), and [^{3}H]propylbenzilylcholine mustards (56) to membrane fractions of the bovine tracheal muscle, the parotid gland, the rat and guinea pig intestine, and the rat, rabbit, and guinea pig heart. They have compared these binding sites to those of the CNS (65). Their findings revealed the presence of virtually identical high-affinity muscarinic cholinergic binding sites in all of the peripheral tissues examined and these receptor sites were quite similar to those of brain. In the heart, for example, the binding sites were stereospecific with dexetimide, the pharmacologically active muscarinic antagonist being 1,000 times more effective in inhibiting [^{3}H]QNB binding than its inactive isomer, levetimide. No inhibition of [^{3}H]QNB binding was produced by nicotinic agents such as α-bungarotoxin and nicotine, indicating the muscarinic specificity of the binding sites. From the above studies it appears that the peripheral muscarinic cholinergic receptors are biochemically similar to those located in the CNS. Further studies will determine whether other neurotransmitter receptors have similar properties in the periphery and in the CNS.

VI. BINDING ASSAY AS A NOVEL CRITERION FOR A NEUROTRANSMITTER

There are several criteria that need to be satisfied in order for a substance to be classified as a neurotransmitter. These criteria include: (a) the presence of the substance in the nerve terminal along with the enzymes required for its biosynthesis and degradation; (b) release of the substance in response to nerve stimulation; (c) similar postsynaptic responses to selective nerve stimulation and to administration of exogenous neurotransmitter; and (d) similar ability of pharmacological agents to interact both with the postsynaptic responses to selective nerve stimulation and with the administration of exogenous substances (62).

In addition to the above criteria, the presence of an appropriate density of neurotransmitter receptors may be thought of as a criterion for identifying a substance as being a neurotransmitter in a given tract or brain region. For example, muscarinic cholinergic receptor density is high in the caudate nucleus and cerebral cortical regions. According to this criterion then, in these brain areas high receptor density suggests that acetylcholine may have a neurotransmitter function. It has been postulated that acetylcholine may be involved in the modulation of movement and in thought processes, respectively in these brain areas (12).

In some brain regions, such as the interpeduncular nucleus, muscarinic receptors are reported to be low in density whereas acetylcholine and its biosynthetic enzyme are reported to be high (34). In such a brain area it is not sufficient to examine only one type of neurotransmitter receptor binding since it is known that acetylcholine can interact with the nicotinic cholinergic receptor as well

(23). In this brain area, it is conceivable that the majority of the receptors are indeed nicotinic.

Another precaution that one will have to consider in the use of this criterion is that neurotransmitter receptor binding may occur where there are no nerve terminals. Specific binding may occur along neuronal axons or to presynaptic elements. Low numbers of specific [^{3}H]nicotine and [^{3}H]QNB binding have been reported in white matter such as the corpus callosum, corona radiata, and cerebral peduncles (16,67). Even with these drawbacks, if proper precautions are taken one may be able to use this criterion as a novel method for identifying a substance as a neurotransmitter when other methods are unavailable.

VII. IDENTIFICATION OF NEUROTRANSMITTER PATHWAYS IN THE BRAIN

Neurotransmitter receptor-binding assays, in conjunction with lesioning methods such as chemical sympathectomy with 6-OHDA, electrolytic lesions, or kainic acid lesions, may provide important information about the neurotransmitter pathways within the CNS. Thus by lesioning specific pathways within the brain one can infer what cell types synapse on the lesioned cells. In addition, information can be gained about the receptor recognition sites and receptor alterations after lesioning.

An example of how lesion studies can be helpful in determining what cell types synapse on the lesioned cell will now be discussed. Coyle and co-workers (13) have reported that intrastriatal injection of kainic acid causes a complete degeneration of neurons intrinsic to the striatum but spares axons of passage and terminals coming from neurons with cell bodies outside the lesioned area. This degeneration is accompanied by severe reduction in neurochemical markers such as glutamic acid decarboxylase (GAD) and choline acetyltransferase (ChAc) located in the striatum. The activity of dopamine-sensitive adenylate cyclase is also dramatically reduced (85%) in the striatum after instrastriatal kainate. Neurotransmitter receptor studies show a 40% reduction in muscarinic cholinergic receptor binding and a 300% increase in GABAergic receptor binding, illustrating that 40% of the cholinergic receptors are localized on cell bodies intrinsic to the striatum whereas GABA receptors may be located on nerve terminals originating from outside of the striatum. Since there is little evidence that muscarinic receptors are associated with glial cells, it seems likely that the remaining 60% of the receptors in the striatum after intrastriatal kainate lesions are associated with axons of passage or with nerve terminals of neurons extrinsic to the striatum. In this respect, recent studies by Westfall (63) indicate that presynaptic muscarinic receptors may regulate the release of dopamine. However, one must be cautious in the interpretation of the binding data. For example, one could have incomplete kainate lesions in the striatum.

Interestingly, when 6-OHDA was injected into the substantia nigra of rats treated with intrastriatal kainate and GABA receptor binding was examined in the striatum, Campochiaro et al. (10) found a significant reduction in GABA binding compared to those animals receiving only intrastriatal kainate, thus indicating that some GABA receptors may be located on nigrostriatal dopamine nerve terminals. From the latter example, one can see that many interesting permutations can be arranged when binding studies are performed in conjunction with lesion studies.

VIII. ALTERATIONS IN NEUROTRANSMITTER RECEPTORS IN NEUROPSYCHIATRIC DISORDERS

During the past few decades a significant amount of information has been accumulated on the biochemistry of synaptic neurotransmission in the human brain; however, relatively few studies have tested for neurotransmitter receptor alterations in this tissue. Since the receptors play a vital role in regulating their own activity either by increasing (supersensitivity) or decreasing (desensitization) their sensitivity to the neurotransmitter, measurements of these receptors may provide valuable clues toward providing rational therapy in diseased states.

A. Receptor Alterations in Huntington's Disease

Huntington's disease (HD) is an autosomal dominant neurological disorder characterized by involuntary choreiform movements and dementia (46). The brain of an adult patient with HD shows marked pathological changes in the basal ganglia, with some neuronal loss occurring in the cerebral cortex and other regions (7). A significant amount of information has accumulated regarding the neurochemical abnormalities of the adult onset form of the disease. As a result of these studies, it seems probable that the most profound neuronal alterations are due to a severe degeneration of neurons that are within the basal ganglia and that utilize acetylcholine and GABA as their neurotransmitters (5,6,20,37,59).

Because of the profound neuronal loss in the basal ganglia in HD, it is possible that the neurotransmitter receptors for dopamine and acetylcholine are destroyed. With the advent of biochemical receptor-binding techniques as described in this book, it is now possible to obtain direct biochemical information concerning the status of these receptors and to design therapeutic protocols accordingly. With this in mind, receptor-binding studies have been undertaken in HD brains (18,19,42,61,68).

Thus far, experiments have shown that the caudate nucleus and putamen of choreic brains show significant reductions in muscarinic cholinergic receptor binding, whereas no significant alterations were observed in other brain regions (61). Significant decreases in dopamine receptor binding were observed in the frontal cortex as well as in the neostriatum (42). Decreases in serotonin binding have also been reported in the neostriatum of HD brain (18,19). The decrease in specific receptor binding in the basal ganglia of HD brain appears to be due to neuronal loss as choline acetyltransferase and GAD activities were also decreased proportionately in the neostriatum of HD brains (19).

One might ask if the decreases in specific ligand binding reflect nonspecific postmortem changes. This is believed to be unlikely since there are no significant decreases in [^{3}H]ligand binding for up to 3 months in frozen intact tissue from rat and monkey brain (19). However, biochemical alterations may occur prior to the freezing of the brain tissue. To examine this, rats were sacrificed and left at room temperature for up to 6 hr prior to removal and freezing of the brain (19). There was no significant difference in the density of the muscarinic cholinergic receptor-binding sites in these rat brains.

Reduction in specific ligand binding in the basal ganglia of HD brain could result from a decreased receptor affinity rather than from a decrease in the density of receptors. This hypothesis was tested by varying the concentrations of [^{3}H]QNB in the binding assay (68). Using the slope from the Scatchard plot, a K_D of approximately 50 pM for the choreic brain was obtained that was not significantly different from the K_D obtained from control human brain. This indicates also that the decrease in specific [^{3}H]QNB binding in HD brain is not due to receptor desensitization. To further insure that the reduction in muscarinic cholinergic binding was due to a decrease in the density of binding sites, the ability of dexetimide, the pharmacologically active stereoisomer of benzetimide, to inhibit [^{3}H]QNB binding in control and HD brains was studied (68). The ability of the active isomer to inhibit [^{3}H]QNB binding was unimpaired.

Further evidence supporting the idea that the decreases in muscarinic cholinergic binding in the basal ganglia is selective, and not due to the result of nonspecific postmortem changes, is the finding that these affected areas are the only areas showing significant decreases in [^{3}H]QNB binding whereas all other brain areas show no changes (61).

Several investigators have previously looked for receptor alterations in the frontal cortex of HD brain; however, no alterations in the density of β-adrenergic, GABAergic, muscarinic cholinergic, or serotonergic receptors were found (19). Recent studies using [^{3}H]spiroperidol to detect dopaminergic receptors have indicated a 65% decrease in [^{3}H]spiroperidol binding within the frontal cortex of HD brains, suggesting that the decrease in receptors may be associated with the neuronal degeneration found in that area (42).

Although Enna et al. (19) did not find significant alterations in [^{3}H]GABA binding in the neostriatum of HD brain, the authors did report (18) finding a significant increase (supersensitivity?) in GABAergic receptors in the substantia nigra of HD brains. Receptor supersensitivity has recently been reported for the β-adrenergic receptors in the rat cerebral cortex after 6-OHDA pretreatment (27).

Cholinomimetic drugs such as oxotremorine, deanol, or choline might be useful in some cases for the symptomatic treatment of HD. These drugs have been administered in HD patients with varying success (15,25,60). Previous clinical trials with the reversible cholinesterase inhibitor physostigmine have been equivocal (32,55). Receptor-binding studies can explain why this may be the case in some patients. Physostigmine nonresponders could represent patients who had severe alterations in the density of striatal muscarinic cholinergic receptors.

B. Receptor Alterations in Parkinson's Disease

Another neurological disorder in which the neurotransmitter receptor has been examined is Parkinson's disease. This disease is a chronic and progressive degenerative disease of the CNS with motor dysfunction due to changes occurring primarily in the nigrostriatal pathway (29). Neurochemically, Parkinson's disease is characterized by a severe deficiency of dopamine and its metabolite, homovanillic acid, within the basal ganglia and the substantia nigra (29). There also seems to be a decrease in tyrosine hydroxylase and dopa decarboxylase activities in this disease (29).

It has been reported that after long-term treatment of Parkinson's disease with L-DOPA, its effectiveness often deteriorates (2,3). For therapy to remain effective some the nigrostriatal dopaminergic neurons as well as their postsynaptic receptors in the basal ganglia must remain intact. The dopaminergic receptor has been examined in Parkinson's disease by the use of the dopaminergic antagonist [^{3}H]spiroperidol (43). A significant (35%) decrease in [^{3}H]spiroperidol binding within the caudate nucleus of parkinsonian brain has been reported (43). From these receptor-binding studies, one could speculate that the loss of effectiveness of L-DOPA therapy after long-term treatment may in part be due to the partial loss of dopaminergic receptors.

C. Other Examples

Mania and depression are two examples of behavioral disorders in which the neurotransmitter receptor-binding sites may be altered within the CNS. Manic–depressive illness is generally characterized by cyclic fluctuation in emotions and behavior (64). It has been postulated that the adrenergic receptor will be supersensitive in the depressive phase due to the lack of an endogenous amine at the synaptic cleft and that the receptor will be subsensitive in the manic phase because of an overabundance of amines at the synaptic junction (8). Although no human brain samples have been studied for neurotransmitter receptor alterations, Banerjee and co-workers (1) have shown that in the rat chronic administration of tricyclic antidepressants that prevent the reuptake of amines into the adrenergic nerve endings produces subsensitivity in the specific binding of [^{3}H]dihydroalprenolol to the β-adrenergic receptor. U'Prichard et al. (57,58) have recently shown that the tricyclic antidepressants may be interacting at the α-adrenergic receptors to produce their antidepressant effect.

Another example in which the receptor may become altered is after chronic treatment with adrenergic stimulants and neuroleptics. Since amphetamine, an adrenergic stimulant, is thought to act by preventing norepinephrine reuptake and also by releasing endogenous norepinephrine from the synaptic terminals (28), it might be predicted that this drug should cause adrenergic subsensitivity. On the other hand, chlorpromazine, a neuroleptic-antipsychotic drug used in the treatment of schizophrenia, may cause dopaminergic receptor supersensitivity upon withdrawal of the drug which may be associated with the production of tardive dyskinesia in humans (33). Studies in the rat model have shown that the neurotransmitter receptor can be modulated to increase after chronic drug administration (9).

A last example where a neurotransmitter receptor binding site may become altered in man may be after traumatic head injury resulting in a specific brain lesion. It is rather difficult to predict receptor alterations occurring under this condition until the exact site of the brain lesion is known. Interestingly, however, specific biochemical and surgical lesions placed in discrete areas of the rat brain have provided valuable information concerning the localization of receptor-binding sites (13,34,66). Rats discretely lesioned with kainic acid or 6-OHDA have provided extremely useful animal models for understanding the neurochemical alterations in such disorders at Huntington's chorea and tardive dyskinesia, respectively (9,13).

IX. SUMMARY

Possible ways in which neurotransmitter receptor-binding assays can be used to answer a number of neurobiological and pharmacological questions about the nervous system have been discussed. For example, it is possible to study the relationship between pre- and postsynaptic receptor development. Prior to the existence of biochemical assays for receptors, it was virtually impossible to directly study this issue.

Another important use of the receptor-binding assays is determining the presence of presynaptic neurotransmitter receptors. Binding techniques used in conjunction with electrolytic or chemical lesioning methods could provide valuable information about the characteristics of these receptors in nervous tissue.

Other questions such as the similarity between central and peripheral neurotransmitter receptors, and the existence of spare receptors can be answered using receptor-binding techniques. Neurotransmitter-binding assays may also be used as a criterion for neurotransmitter identification, and the assay can be used to help identify neurotransmitter pathways within the brain.

Receptor-binding studies performed on neurologically diseased brains should yield information about the status of the receptor that may be helpful in suggesting a therapeutic treatment.

ACKNOWLEDGMENT

Preparation of the manuscript was facilitated by grants from the following sources: USPHS MH–27257, MH–30626, the Huntington's Chorea Foundation.

The author is a recipient of a Research Scientist Development Award (RSDA) from the NIMH (MH–00095).

X. REFERENCES

1. Banerjee, S. P., Kung, L. S., Riggi, S. J., and Chanda, S. K. (1977): Development of β-adrenergic receptor subsensitivity by antidepressants. *Nature (Lond),* 268:455–456.
2. Barbeau, A. (1976): Six years of high-level levodopa therapy in severely akinetic parkinsonian patients. *Arch. Neurol.,* 33:333–338.
3. Barbeau, A., and Roy, M. (1976): Six-year results of treatment with levodopa plus benzerazide in Parkinson's disease. *Neurology (Minneap),* 26:399–404.
4. Beld, A. J., Van Den Hoven, S., Wouterse, A. C., and Zegers, M. A. P. (1975): Are muscarinic receptors in the central and peripheral nervous system different? *Eur. J. Pharmacol.,* 30:360–363.
5. Bird, E. D., and Iversen, L. L. (1974): Huntington's chorea: Post-mortem measurement of glutamic acid decarboxylase, choline acetyltransferase and dopamine in basal ganglia. *Brain,* 97:457–472.
6. Bird, E. D., and Iversen, L. L. (1976): Neurochemical findings in Huntington's chorea. In: *Essays in Neurochemistry and Neuropharmacology,* edited by M. Youdim, D. Sharman, W. Lovenberg, and J. Ragnodo, pp. 177–195. Wiley, New York.
7. Blackwood, W., McMenemey, W. H., Meyer, A., Norman, R. M., and Russell, D. S. (1967): *Greenfields' Neuropathology,* pp. 553–558. Williams & Wilkins, Baltimore.
8. Bunny, W. E. (1978): Psychopharmacology of the switch process in affective illness. In: *Psychopharmacology: A Generation of Progress,* edited by M. A. Lipton, A. DiMascio, and K. F. Killiam, pp. 1249–1259. Raven Press, New York.
9. Burt, D. R., Creese, I., and Snyder, S. H. (1977): Antischizophrenic drugs: Chronic treatment elevates dopamine receptor binding in brain. *Science,* 196:326–328.
10. Campochiaro, P., Schwarcz, R., and Coyle, J. T. (1977): GABA receptor binding in rat striatum: Localization and effect of denervation. *Brain Res.,* 136:501–511.
11. Carlsson, A., Kehr, N., Lindquist, M., Magnusson, T., and Atack, C. (1972): Regulation of monoamine metabolism in the central nervous system. *Pharmacol. Rev.,* 24:371–384.
12. Coyle, J. T., and Yamamura, H. I. (1976): Neurochemical aspects of the ontogenesis of cholinergic neurons in the rat brain. *Brain Res.,* 118:429–440.
13. Coyle, J. T., Schwarcz, R., Bennett, J. P., and Campochiaro, P. (1977): Clinical, neuropathologic and pharmacologic aspects of Huntington's disease: Correlates with a new animal model. *Prog. Neuropsychopharmacol.,* 1:13–30.
14. Creese, I., and Snyder, S. H. (1975): Receptor binding and pharmacological activity of opiates in the guinea pig intestine. *J. Pharmacol. Exp. Ther.,* 194:205–219.
15. Davis, K. L., Hollister, L. E., Barchas, J. P., and Berger, P. A. (1976): Choline in tardive dyskinesia and Huntington's disease. *Life Sci.,* 19:1507–1516.
16. Denberg, J. L., and O'Brien, R. D. (1973): Axonal cholinergic binding macromolecule: Response to neuroactive drugs. *J. Med. Chem.,* 16:57–60.
17. Diamond, J., and Miledi, R. (1962): A study of fetal and newborn rat muscle fibers. *J. Physiol. (Lond),* 162:393–408.
18. Enna, S. J., Bennett, J. P., Bylund, D. B., Snyder, S. H., Bird, E. D., and Iversen, L. L. (1976): Alterations of brain neurotransmitter receptor binding in Huntington's chorea. *Brain Res.,* 116:531–536.
19. Enna, S. J., Bird, E. D., Bennett, J. P., Bylund, D. B., Yamamura, H. I., Iversen, L. L., and Snyder, S. H. (1976): Huntington's chorea: Changes in neurotransmitter receptors in the brain. *N. Engl. J. Med.,* 294:1305–1309.
20. Enna, S. J., Stern, L. Z., Wastek, G. J., and Yamamura, H. I. (1977): Neurobiology and pharmacology of Huntington's disease. *Life Sci.,* 23:205–212.
21. Farnebo, L-O., and Hamberger, B. (1970): Effects of desipramine, phentolamine and phenoxybenzamine on the release of noradrenaline from isolated tissues, *J. Pharm. Pharmacol.,* 22:855–857.
22. Fields, J. Z., Roeske, W. R., Morkin, E., and Yamamura, H. I. (1978): Demonstration of muscarinic cholinergic binding in the mammalian heart. *J. Biol. Chem.,* 253:3251–3257.

23. Fishbach, G. D., and Cohen, S. A. (1973): The distribution of acetylcholine sensitivity over uninnervated and innervated muscle fibers grown in cell cultures. *Dev. Biol.,* 31:147–162.
24. Furchgott, R. F. (1964): Receptor mechanisms. *Annu. Rev. Pharmacol.,* 4:21–50.
25. Growdon, J. H., Cohen, E. L., and Wurtman, R. J. (1977): Huntington's disease: Clinical and chemical effects on choline administration, *Ann. Neurol.,* 1:418–422.
26. Harden, T. K., Wolfe, B. B., Sporn, J. R., Perkins, J. P., and Molinoff, P. B. (1977): Ontogeny of β-adrenergic receptors in rat cerebral cortex. *Brain Res.,* 125:99–108.
27. Harden, T. K., Wolfe, B. B., Sporn, J. R., Poulos, B. K., and Molinoff, P. B. (1977): Effects of 6-hydroxydopamine on the development of the β-adrenergic receptor/adenylate cyclase system in rat cerebral cortex. *J. Pharmacol. Exp. Ther.,* 203:132–143.
28. Horn, A. S., Coyle, J. T., and Snyder, S. H. (1971): Catecholamine uptake by synaptosomes from rat brain: Structure-activity relationships of drugs with differential effects on dopamine and norepinephrine neurons. *Mol. Pharmacol.,* 7:66–80.
29. Hornykiewicz, O. (1975): Parkinson's disease and its chemotherapy. *Biochem. Pharmacol.,* 24:1061–1065.
30. Johnson, G. A., and Mitchell, J. F. (1971): The effect of bicuculline, metrazol, picrotoxin and strychnine on the release of ^{3}H-GABA from rat brain slices. *J. Neurochem.,* 18:2441–2446.
31. Kirpekar, S. M., and Puig, M. (1971): Effect of flow-stop on noradrenaline release from normal spleens and spleens treated with cocaine, phentolamine or phenoxybenzamine. *Br. J. Pharmacol.,* 43:359–369.
32. Klawans, H. L., and Rubovits, R. (1972): Central cholinergic-anticholinergic antagonism in Huntington's chorea. *Neurology (Minneap),* 22:107–116.
33. Kobayashi, R. M. (1976): Orofacial dyskinesia-clinical features, mechanisms and drug therapy. *West. J. Med.,* 125:277–288.
34. Kuhar, M. J., DeHaven, R. N., Yamamura, H. I., Rommelspacher, H., and Simon, J. R. (1975): Further evidence for cholinergic habenulo-interpeduncular neurons: Pharmacologic and functional characteristics. *Brain Res.,* 97:265–275.
35. Kuhar, M. J., Sethy, V. H., Roth, R. H., and Aghajanian, G. K. (1973): Choline: Selective accumulation by central cholinergic neurons. *J. Neurochem.,* 20:581–593.
36. Lewis, P. R., and Shute, C. C. D. (1967): The cholinergic limbic system. *Brain,* 90:521–540.
37. McGeer, P. L., and McGeer, E. G. (1976): Enzymes associated with the metabolism of catecholamines, acetylcholine and GABA in human controls and patients with Parkinson's disease and Huntington's chorea. *J. Neurochem.,* 26:65–76.
38. Mitchell, J. F. (1963): The spontaneous and evoked release of acetylcholine from the cerebral cortex, *J. Physiol. (Lond),* 165:98–116.
39. Molenaar, P. C., and Polak, R. L. (1970): Stimulation by atropine of acetylcholine release and synthesis in cortical slices from rat brain. *Br. J. Pharmacol.,* 40:406–417.
40. Mohler, H., and Okada, T. (1977): Benzodiazepine receptor: Demonstration in the central nervous system. *Science,* 198:849–851.
41. Polak, R. L., and Meeuws, M. M. (1966): The influence of atropine on the release and uptake of acetylcholine by the isolated cerebral cortex of the rat. *Biochem. Pharmacol.,* 15:989–992.
42. Reisine, T. D., Fields, J. Z., Stern, L. Z., Johnson, P. C., Bird, E. D., and Yamamura, H. I. (1977): Alterations in dopaminergic receptors in Huntington's disease. *Life Sci.,* 21:1123–1128.
43. Reisine, T. D., Fields, J. Z., Yamamura, H. I., Bird, E. D., Spokes, E., Schreiner, P. S., and Enna, S. J. (1977): Neurotransmitter receptor alterations in Parkinson's disease. *Life Sci.,* 21:335–344.
44. Roeske, W. R., and Yamamura, H. I. (1978): Maturation of mammalian myocardial muscarinic cholinergic receptors. *Life Sci. (in press).*
45. Sharma, V. K., and Banerjee, S. P. (1977): Presynaptic muscarinic cholinergic receptors in rat heart sympathetic nerves. *Eur. J. Pharmacol.,* 46:75–76.
46. Shoulson, I., and Chase, T. N. (1975): Huntington's disease. *Annu. Rev. Med.,* 26:419–426.
47. Snyder, S. H., Banerjee, S. P., Yamamura, H. I., and Greenberg, D. (1974): Drugs, neurotransmitters and schizophrenia. *Science,* 184:1243–1253.
48. Speth, R., Wastek, G. J., Johnson, P. C., and Yamamura, H. I. (1978): Benzodiazepine binding in human brain: Characterization using ^{3}H-flunitrazepam. *Life Sci.,* 22:859–866.
49. Squires, R., and Braestrup, C. (1977): Benzodiazepine receptors in rat brain. *Nature (Lond),* 266:732–734.

50. Starke, K. (1971): Influence of α-receptor stimulants on noradrenaline release. *Naturwissenschaften,* 58:420–425.
51. Starke, K. (1973): Influence of extracellular noradrenaline on the stimulation evoked secretion of noradrenaline from sympathetic nerves: Evidence for an α-receptor-mediated feed-back inhibition of noradrenaline release. *Naunym Schmiedebergs Arch. Exp. Path. Pharmac.,* 275:11–23.
52. Starke, K., Montel, H. and Wagner, J. (1971): Effect of phentolamine on noradrenaline uptake and release. *Naunyn-Schmiedeberg's Arch. Pharmacol.,* 271:181–192.
53. Szerb, J. C. (1978): The characterization of presynaptic muscarinic receptors in central cholinergic neurons. In: *Cholinergic Mechanisms and Psychopharmacology,* edited by D. J. Jenden, pp. 49–60. Plenum Press, New York.
54. Szerb, J. C., and Somogyi, G. T. (1973): Depression of acetylcholine release from cerebral cortical slices by cholinesterase inhibition and by oxotremorine. *Nature* [*New Biol.*], 241:121–122.
55. Tarsy, D., Leopold, N., and Sax, D. X. (1974): Physostigmine in choreiform movement disorders. *Neurology (Minneap),* 24:28–33.
56. Taylor, I. K., Cuthbert, A. W., and Young, J. M. (1975): Muscarinic receptors in rat intestinal muscle: Comparison with the guinea pig. *Eur. J. Pharmacol.,* 31:319–326.
57. U'Prichard, D. C., and Snyder, S. H. (1977): Therapeutic and side effects of psychotropic drugs: The relevance of receptor binding methodology. In: *Animal Models in Psychiatry and Neurology,* edited by I. Hanin and E. Usdin, pp. 477–495, Pergamon Press, New York.
58. U'Prichard, D. C., Greenberg, D. A., Sheehan, P. P., and Snyder, S. H. (1978): Tricyclic antidepressants: Therapeutic properties and affinity for α-noradrenergic receptor binding sites in the brain. *Science,* 199:197–198.
59. Urquhart, N., Perry, T. L., Hansen, S., and Kennedy, J. (1975): GABA content and glutamic acid decarboxylase activity in brain of Huntington's chorea patients and control subjects. *J. Neurochem.,* 24:1071–1075.
60. Walker, J. E., Hoehn, M., Sears, E., and Lewis, J. (1973): Dimethylaminoethanol in Huntington's chorea. *Lancet,* 1:1512–1513.
61. Wastek, G. J., Stern, L. Z., Johnson, P. C., and Yamamura, H. I. (1976): Huntington's disease: Regional alterations in muscarinic cholinergic receptor binding in human brain. *Life Sci.,* 19:1033–1040.
62. Werman, R. (1966): Criteria for identification of a central nervous system transmitter. *Comp. Biochem. Physiol.,* 18:745–766.
63. Westfall, T. (1974): Effect of muscarinic agonists on the release of ^{3}H-norepinephrine and ^{3}H-dopamine by potassium and electrical stimulation from rat brain slices. *Life Sci.,* 14:1641–1652.
64. Winokur, G. (1978): Mania and depression: family studies and genetics in relation to treatment. In: *Psychopharmacology: A Generation of Progress,* edited by M. A. Lipton, A. DiMascio, and K. F. Killiam, pp. 1213–1221. Raven Press, New York.
65. Yamamura, H. I., and Snyder, S. H. (1974): Muscarinic cholinergic binding in rat brain. *Proc. Natl. Acad. Sci. USA,* 71:1725–1729.
66. Yamamura, H. I., and Snyder, S. H. (1974): Postsynaptic localization of muscarcinic cholinergic receptor binding in rat hippocampus. *Brain Res.,* 78:320–326.
67. Yamamura, H. I., Kuhar, M. J., Greenberg, D., and Snyder, S. H. (1974): Muscarinic cholinergic binding: Regional distribution in monkey brain. *Brain Res.,* 66:541–546.
68. Yamamura, H. I., Wastek, G. J., Johnson, P. C., and Stern, L. Z. (1978): Biochemical characterization of muscarinic cholinergic receptors in Huntington's disease. In: *Cholinergic Mechanisms and Psychopharmacology* edited by D. J. Jenden, pp. 35–47. Plenum Press, New York.

SUBJECT INDEX

Subject Index